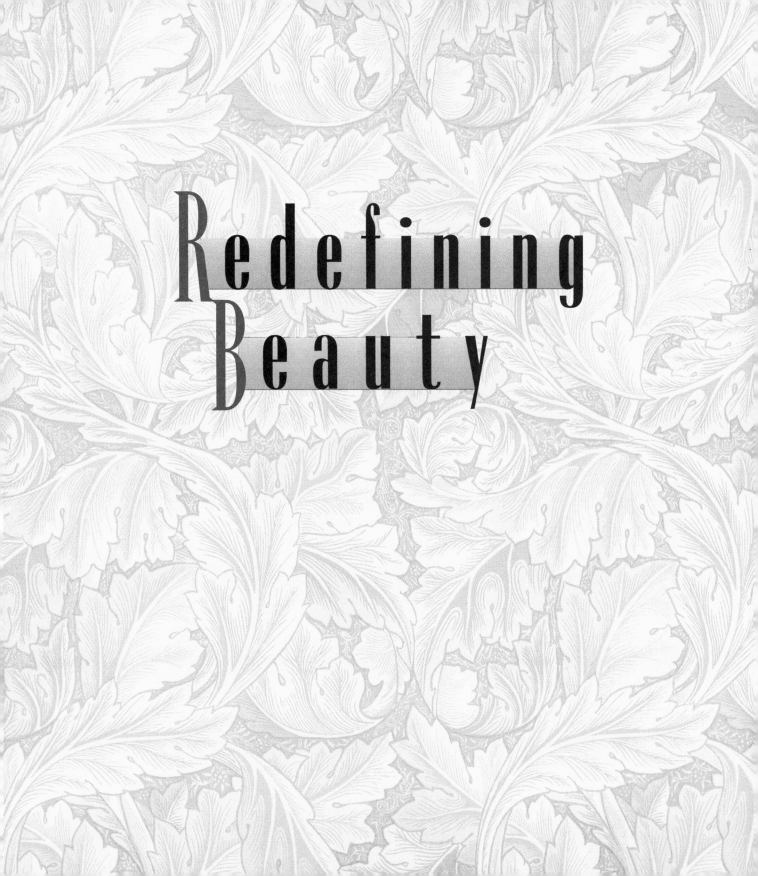

Redefining Beauty

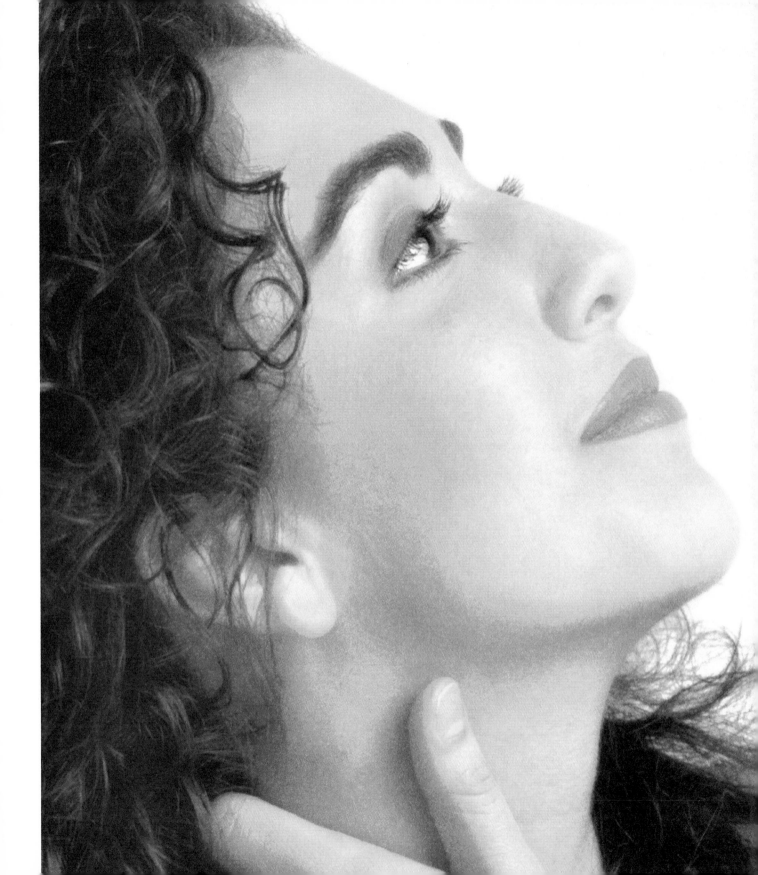

Redefining Beauty

Discovering your individual beauty, enhancing your self-esteem

Victoria Jackson

with Paddy Calistro
Photography by Douglas Kirkland

Book design by Michaelis/Carpelis Design

WARNER BOOKS

A Time Warner Company

Warner Books, Inc.
1271 Avenue of the Americas, New York, NY 10020

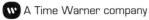 A Time Warner company

Printed in the United States of America
First Printing: November 1993
10 9 8 7 6 5 4 3 2 1

Library of Congress Cataloging-in-Publication Data

Jackson, Victoria.
    Redefining beauty: discovering your individual beauty,
    enhancing your self-esteem/Victoria Jackson with Paddy Calistro.
    p. cm.
    ISBN 0-446-51740-2
    1. Body image. 2. Beauty, Personal–Psychological aspects.
    3. Cosmetics–Psychological aspects. 4. Self-esteem.
I. Calistro, Paddy.
II. Title.

BF697,5.B63J33 1993
646,7'042–dc20
                                         92-51032
                                         CIP

Photography by Douglas Kirkland
Book design by Michaelis/Carpelis Design

DEDICATION

To women the world over whose positive spirit

inspired me. Their faith in themselves

has encouraged and validated my belief

that every woman is beautiful.

ACKNOWLEDGMENTS

Although I have always dreamed of sharing my thoughts on beauty in a book, I never would have ventured farther without the support of so many wonderful people. I am especially grateful to my husband, Bill Guthy, for urging me to put my ideas on paper—his love and support kept me going. My thanks, too, to Joe Minogue, for his encouragement during the early years of my career as a makeup artist. A special loving thank-you to my son, Evan, who always keeps me laughing. And thanks to my little daughter, Alexandra Rose, who patiently waited to be born until this book was completed. My gratitude to my brother Dan, who had so much faith in his sister and has always been so supportive. And to my mom, who still helps maintain some order in my life; I'm always grateful that she told me to wash my face and put on some makeup during those formative years.

The makeup demonstrated so beautifully in this book is the work of my colleague and friend, makeup artist Denise Landau, whom I first encountered when she enrolled in the makeup classes I taught at UCLA so many years ago; she is the ultimate professional. Credit must go, too, to Mickey Song, whose artistry with hair complements the women you'll meet in these pages; his positive attitude is contagious.

It is an honor to work with photographer Douglas Kirkland. His work clearly and honestly portrays the natural beauty of each of the women featured throughout this book. When he's behind the camera, I'm always confident that I'll look my very best. His support and encouragement were a constant motivation to me during my years as a makeup artist.

The beautiful women in Douglas's photographs deserve a special thank-you. Each of them was lovely when we started and even lovelier as the days wore on. They are the heart and soul of my book.

Maureen Mahon Egen, the publisher of Warner Hardcover Books, immediately recognized the importance of redefining beauty. Her positive spirit and belief in the project made the process a pleasure.

Many thanks to Irene Carpelis and Sylvain Michaelis of Michaelis/Carpelis, for the inspired graphic design and visual excitement on every page.

My gratitude, too, to Mel Berger, Rick Bradley, and Rick Hersh of the William Morris Agency for their dedication to the project. Much appreciation goes to John Marsh, Steve Scott, Jim Shaughnessy, Karen Heft, and the support team at American Telecast Corporation; without their confidence in me there would be no Victoria Jackson Cosmetics. I will always be grateful that they recognized the potential in my ideas and my products.

Much appreciation goes to two special friends, Judy Zegarelli and Daina Hulet, whose support is a wonderful force in my life.

Donna Pregler and Anne Hamilton deserve special thanks for their abiding energy and attention to detail.

Finally, my gratitude to my friend, Paddy Calistro, who took my thoughts and turned them into all the right words. I had a dream; she helped me make it happen.

Victoria

TABLE OF CONTENTS

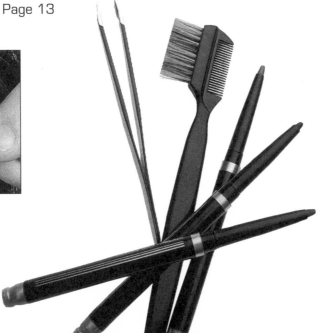
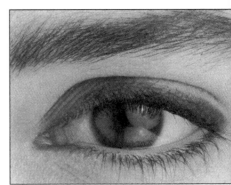

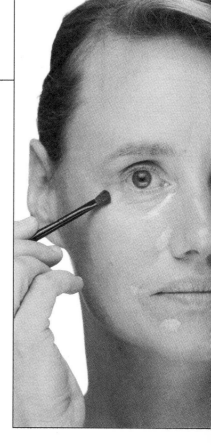

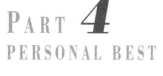

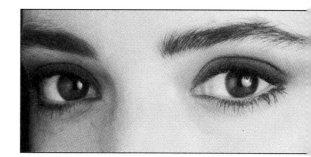

Introduction

When I looked in the mirror a couple of years ago, I saw myself—I mean, I really saw myself. Sure, there was the same Victoria Jackson I knew ten years ago—the eyes were still brown, the nose a little crooked, the uneven lips, the complexion nice and clear. But suddenly I saw things that weren't apparent a decade ago: in addition to a few extra laugh lines, there—to my surprise—was my success, my knowledge, my experience, the man I love, my children. Reflected in the mirror was the story of my life, the happy days, the crazy days, the relentless days. And I realized I was looking at a beautiful woman. And I liked her very much.

That was a turning point for me. My years as a Hollywood makeup artist had taught me to look at other people and immediately see their true beau-

> **❝Zest is the secret of all beauty. There is no beauty that is attractive without zest.❞**
>
> —Christian Dior

> **❝The image of woman as we know it is an image created by men and fashioned to suit their needs.❞**
>
> —Kate Millett

ty, but for whatever reasons I was a lot harder on myself. In those days my self-esteem was at its lowest. When I looked in the mirror I hated the reflection. Because I didn't look like a movie star or the cover girl of the day, I never quite measured up. No angular face, no big blue eyes, no prominent cheekbones. I was buying into the definitions of beauty that I had seen in cosmetics advertisements and on TV and in film.

Occasionally there would be a revelation. Like the day I was assigned to work on Bette Davis's face, shortly before she died. I had heard all the horror stories about her being vain and difficult, so I had prepared myself mentally for a difficult day. As I started to apply foundation on that wrinkled skin, she stared at me with those determined eyes and then put her hand on mine to stop my progress. "Don't use all that makeup to try to cover my lines, honey," she ordered. "I've earned every single one of them." It was an important lesson for me. She had learned to accept her face as the symbol of her success.

> **"The most beautiful makeup of a woman is a passion. But cosmetics are easier to buy."**
>
> —Yves Saint Laurent

> **"Though we travel the world over to find the beautiful, we must carry it with us or we find it not."**
>
> —Ralph Waldo Emerson

Those wrinkles were part of her life. As I looked at her—lines and all—I suddenly saw an incredible ageless beauty.

The experience gave me a new take on aging. In my work I then was able to start looking at a woman's face and not strive to make her appear "younger"—my goal was to enhance her honestly. I wanted every woman, no matter what her age, to demonstrate that ageless, timeless quality I had seen in Miss Davis's face.

But I soon realized that only a few of the beautiful women I met each day could accept their own natural appearance. Most of them had been programmed to hide behind masks of makeup. I was never very comfortable when asked to drastically change a woman's appearance. My personal choice was to enhance her natural beauty, to

> **"Beauty—the adjustment of all parts proportionately so that one cannot add or subtract or change without impairing the harmony of the whole."**
>
> —Leon Battista Alberti

make her look like herself, only better.

My signature has always been "no-makeup makeup"—I've spent years showing women how to look natural. Once a woman sees her own special beauty with makeup, it's much easier for her to appreciate her face with no makeup.

When I think of the embodiment of the natural look, I immediately picture Ali MacGraw. As any of you who watch my TV shows know, we've been friends for years, and not just because she wears my cosmetics. It was Ali who urged me to start marketing my foundation—she believed in me that much. But despite the fact that she loves my products, she's just as apt to go out barefaced as with makeup on. She seems perfectly at ease either way, and she has for as long as I've known her. The first time I met her she strolled into the photo studio with just a slick of lipstick on her lips and no other makeup. That was a dozen years ago. Today she still looks and feels great when she's barefaced.

"When the candles are out all women are fair."

—Plutarch

As the title of this book says, I'm here to redefine beauty, to lift the limits, expand the parameters...whatever it takes. On the following pages you will see women of many ages, colorations, and ethnic heritages. These women represent the essence of true beauty. Each one of them has unique features and a unique personality that add up to her individual beauty.

By the time you finish this book, I want you to look in the mirror and love yourself and your face. Sure, I'll teach you how to use makeup to enhance your natural looks, but I don't want you to think in terms of changing. I like your face the way it is, and I hope you do, too. There's no reason to strive to alter your image to match someone else's. I urge you not to try to adapt to someone else's perception of beauty. Instead I encourage you to strive to raise your self-esteem, to discover your individual beauty, to enhance it, and, above all, to cherish it.

"As a white candle In a holy place, So is the beauty Of an aged face."

—Joseph Campbell

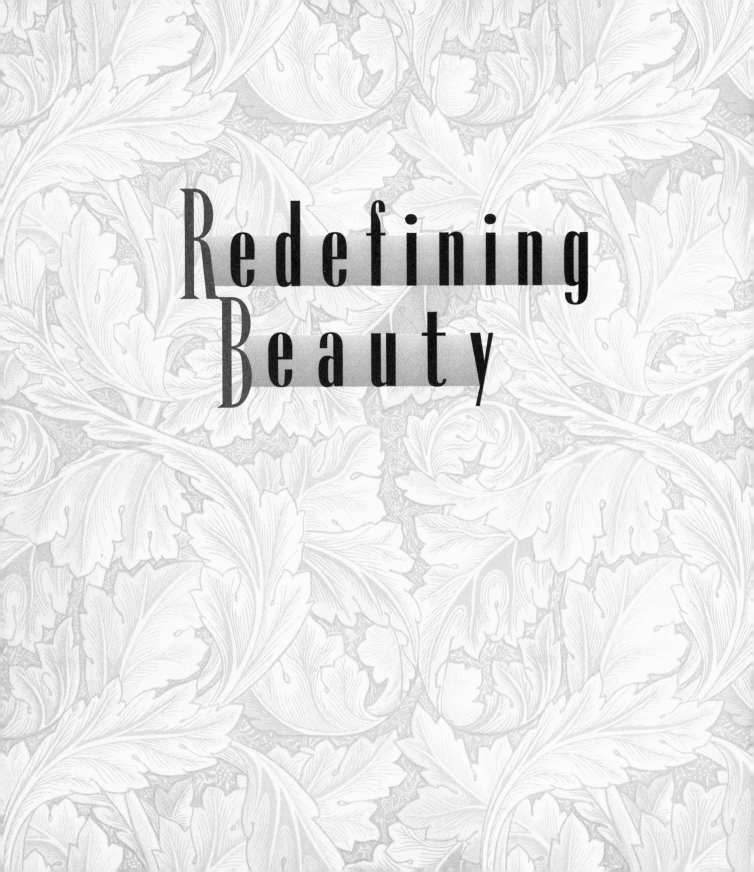

Redefining Beauty

Making Sense of Beauty

*Nice as it is on the surface, "beautiful"
has always been a threatening word.
It's like "perfect," a word that always
refers to someone or something else,
not us. We've all looked in the mirror,
observed a face that didn't measure up
to the current standards of beauty and
we've ended up feeling lousy. We've got
to change our perspective. We must
look at ourselves and feel fantastic.
And we can!*

You Don't Need to Wear Makeup

Repeat after me: "I don't need to wear makeup. I'm beautiful without it. I don't need to wear makeup. I'm beautiful without it." I know—you think I must be crazy. After all, I am the chairman of the board of a cosmetics company. If every woman gave up wearing makeup, I'd be out of business. But, if every woman looked in the mirror and felt truly beautiful and truly good about herself, the trade-off would be worth it.

That's why that affirmation is so important to me. You don't need makeup; I don't need makeup. We are beautiful without it. I want to dispel any notion that makeup is the reason for our good looks. I repeat, we are beautiful without it. When you can see your face stripped of all makeup and be comfortable with your eyes, nose, lips, chin, cheeks, brows, and face shape, you will have discovered your own honest beauty. You'll be able to go out on the street barefaced with confidence.

My goal, of course, is not for you to throw away your lipstick and mascara—mine or any other brand. I want you to enjoy makeup as much as I do, without feeling enslaved to it. Makeup is one of the many positive aspects of being female. In fact, there are about 100 pages of this book devoted entirely to to the application of cosmetics. Obviously I believe that makeup offers a great deal. The assets go on and on: You can use it to enhance everything that's beautiful about you. It's fun. It's a small indulgence that boosts your spirits. People regard you differently when you wear it. You don't have to be a certain size or shape to look great in it. You can take it anywhere. Girlfriends can gab about it for hours. It has no calories. It hides those dark circles that develop after staying up all night. If you get sick of it, soap and water dissolves it. Best of all, you're in total control of it (or you will be, by the time you follow the steps in this book).

Notice that I did not say that it will change your life. Makeup doesn't make love happen. Nor does wearing it make you rich and famous. You won't get a promotion by changing your lipstick. Nor does it de-age you or your skin. Wrinkles won't fade away, and even little sags won't firm up. (All that hope-in-a-jar baloney is just that.)

Note, too, that makeup won't make you love yourself. But if you want to boost your self-esteem and you're willing to take some action in that direction, applying some lipstick and blush will help. To some of you that may sound shallow and simplistic at first. It isn't. As you read on, I hope you'll be convinced that I view makeup simply as a step toward self-acceptance. Wearing natural-looking makeup will help make a difference in how you feel about yourself. Maybe it's because seeing a brighter face in the mirror is like seeing a bright sky—subliminally uplifting. Or perhaps it's because highlighting your natural features confirms how nice they are to begin with. Maybe it's because wearing makeup helps you reach your image potential, and that gives you the impetus to attempt reaching more important goals. Or maybe the answer is even more straightforward: devoting a little extra attention to yourself feels good. I can't explain why it works: I just know it does.

I've seen makeup make a difference time and time again. There have been days in my own life when I was really down, days when it seemed impossible that anything could go the way I wanted. Lacking a better solution, I remembered the advice my mother always gave me when I was a teenager: "Wash your face, comb your hair, and put on some makeup." No situations changed. But my clean face and some color made me feel that I looked better. That positive feeling improved my outlook, and somehow I made it through. At least I knew that I looked my best, which gave me more confidence and, at the worst of times, a bit of hope. (Obviously it's no coincidence that I became a makeup artist!)

Granted, I'm no psychologist (nor would I want to be), but I have often observed the dramatic link between accepting our physical image and a strong self-image. I can also assure you that people who feel positively about the person they see in the mirror have more success than those who don't. I've seen that proven repeatedly in the two self-esteem programs I founded, one for cancer patients at Cedars-Sinai Medical Center and another for prisoners ready to be released at the Sybil Brand Institute for women in Los Angeles.

In both places I meet women with depleted egos, women who need a helping hand, women who simply want to feel better. I teach them easy makeup techniques that can help change the first impression they make when they meet others. The first thing I do is show them how attractive they are without makeup, even though they've been ravaged by chemotherapy or prison life. Then I demonstrate how adding some natural-looking color will enhance their unique features and help them attain a healthier glow. I've watched many of them go on to take control of their lives, actively beating their odds. No, wearing makeup didn't change their lives: they did. But accepting the reality of their physical images, feeling confident about their looks, and experiencing other people's positive response to them gave them the boost they needed to start exercising their personal power and making those big breakthroughs.

I'm constantly struck by examples of the relationship between good grooming and feeling better about ourselves. Several doctors have told me that when a woman is recovering in the hospital, a reliable indicator that she's feeling better is when she begins putting on her makeup and brushing her hair. And very often someone who's dieting will admit that she got a haircut or bought new lipstick even before she purchased new clothes. Turning to makeup is a common response—a small but reassuring step. In these instances people are caring for themselves again after a period when they couldn't find the physical or emotional strength to do something positive.

I was initially inspired to write this book by the hundreds of letters I've received from clients who wanted to share with me some of the pivotal moments in their lives. I want to offer a few of their stories to you. Yes, the letters all refer to using my products, but makeup was just the catalyst for writing to me. I really believe that these women began caring about their looks at a significant point in their lives, a time when they needed a jump-start to increase their self-esteem. Each of them took the initiative to find a tool that would provide that extra push. In their cases, it was makeup. But the women made the changes they describe, not the products. This first letter shows how one woman elevated her self-confidence after a long battle to save her husband's life:

I am a 23-year-old mother, wife, and businesswoman. All that I love was almost lost on August 16, 1990. While vacationing, my husband was critically burned over 50 percent of his body. By the grace of God he survived. After 3 months he was discharged from the hospital and needed my 24-hour care, so I was unable to go back to work. He improved and I finally went back, but not before getting your products. I needed a lift to help recapture some of the youthful looks I had lost. I think my co-workers were expecting to see an emotionally and physically distraught woman. What a surprise when I walked in with a confident smile and a beautiful glow.

— J.M., Greenbelt, Maryland

J.M.'s letter commands such respect. Her self-sacrifice for the man she loved was remarkable and surely saved his life. Then, when she realized that she had lost some of her self-confidence by lovingly devoting so much time and energy to his recovery, she knew what she had to do. Consider her circumstances: she was walking into a room filled with people who were ready to feel sorry for her, she hadn't had the opportunity for much outside conversation, she had survived a devastating tragedy, finances were tight after all the medical expenses, and she was worried about how her husband would feel when she went back to the workplace. At the right stage in his convalescence, she knew that her return to work was the necessary step and that a little superficial lift would make the first day easier. People at work responded to that happy, healthy face, and a cycle of renewal began.

The next letter is from a woman who also used makeup as a confidence builder.

In October of 1990 I got laid off from the job that I had for over 2 years. In January 1991 I finally got a chance to interview for a great new job. Before I went on that interview I made myself look the best I possibly could. I used your makeup the way you had taught me, and I felt very assured, because when you look and feel your best, it presents a better picture of you. I knew with the proper makeup I was presenting a professional image that was needed to get the job I wanted. One week later I got the job, and I owe it to my new image and self-confidence.

— D.N., Billings, Montana

Like it or not, people do judge you by how you look. Knowing that, D.N. presented herself as professionally as she would her résumé That first impression lasts only for a minute, of course, but that's enough time for a prospective employer to evaluate your self-respect, self-confidence, and sense of propriety. Someone who walks into a job with no makeup whatsoever may put across a less refined image than another person who is tastefully groomed, wearing an appropriate amount of makeup. D.N. put careful thought into each phase of her presentation—her ideas, her salesmanship, her image. It paid off.

T.F. tells a story to which many women can relate. She was making the break back into a career after being a busy young mother:

In the fall of '89 I began teaching full-time after 4 years of raising my two boys. I had gained weight and was not in the habit of dressing up every day. I purchased your makeup and began experimenting. I started getting compliments and feeling better. I started a dance class, lost weight, and then started caring for my skin. Relatives said I looked years younger. I felt years younger. Then the best: when I attended my 20-year eighth-grade class reunion, I was voted the person "least changed." Thank you for helping me regain a lot of lost confidence.

—T.F., Lake St. Louis, Missouri

In many ways the letters from T.F. and J.M. tell similar stories, though one is based in near tragedy and one in the joy of raising children. As T.F. raised her sons and J.M. cared for her suffering husband, both women forgot about themselves because they were so involved in their love for others. How interesting that both of them considered makeup as the little boost that would get them started. They knew what they needed and took the initiative to use it.

What Is Self-Esteem and Why Is a Makeup Expert Talking about It?

Everybody's talking about self-esteem. In fact, "self-esteem" is one of those terms that has become so overused that most of us assume we know the meaning—yet when asked to define it, we stumble, searching for the right words. In my old edition of Webster's dictionary, "self-esteem" is aptly wedged midway between "self-doubt" and "self-expression." Its definition reads: "belief in oneself; self-respect." Most psychologists have expanded the meaning to include such terms as "self-confidence" and "pride." On the surface the words are so common, yet they hold the essence of our being. Our belief in ourselves, our self-respect, our self-confidence, and our pride—what are we without them?

As we all know, self-esteem can be high (we feel good about ourselves) or low (we feel inadequate). Psychologists say that almost every aspect of our lives—our personal happiness, success, relationships with others, achievement, creativity, dependencies, even our sex lives—are dependent on our level of self-esteem. The more we have, the better we deal with things.

What we sometimes forget is that we are all capable of increasing our self-esteem, no matter how high or low we may feel on any given day. The good feelings we can generate about ourselves are limitless. Most important, these feelings are within our control, independent of how the rest of the world views us. What that means in the context of this book is that I can go on for pages telling you how wonderful and beautiful you are, but until you believe it, your self-esteem will be low. (I'm hopeful that reading this book will help you to discover ways to increase your self-esteem, however!) Another person may guess from observing you and your reactions that you are a wonderful, beautiful woman with low self-esteem, but only you know if she's correct. Only you know how much self-respect, self-confidence, and pride is welling up inside you...or is buried too deep to feel.

I only wish that putting on makeup would be the single key to immediately raising women's self-esteem. No such magic. In fact, in the past many cosmetics advertisements and cosmetics themselves have contributed to women's lowered self-esteem. People buy nearly $20 billion worth of cosmetics each year because they consciously or subconsciously think they need them. The beauty industry has hammered away at us that it's wrong to look older than 25. It has misled us with 18-year-old faces advertising antiaging creams and convinced us that artifice somehow makes us more beautiful and appealing than we already are. To me that's a misuse of power.

The first—and most important—step in building self-esteem is to accept ourselves before we attempt to improve. There's something very wrong when an entire industry is coercing us into trying to be different from who we are. I went into the beauty business because I like the way makeup helps women look their best. I wanted to simplify everything about its application and strip away the negative mystique. I knew from the beginning that if makeup didn't intimidate women, they would get the most from it. That's why I began spreading what, for me, is the most important message about makeup: it's a tool to make us look and feel good.

Used that way, makeup can start a dynamic chain reaction. When you look good, you feel better. When you feel better, you do more. When you do more, you accomplish more. When you accomplish more, your self-confidence zooms. As your self-confidence increases, so does your self-respect. With more self-respect, your overall level of pride increases. And when you have more pride, self-respect, and self-confidence, you can confidently say that you have more self-esteem. You feel more comfortable with yourself.

Makeup is a support that helps start the reaction—the individual takes over immediately through positive action. A well-cared-for physical image provides that final reassurance: "You look great—now go get 'em." With that extra confidence, a woman can forget about how she looks and get on with the rest of her life.

Certainly a hairdresser, exercise teacher, facialist, or clothing designer could spread the same message with regard to each specialty. A new hairstyle, an active workout, a well-tended complexion, or a great new outfit can each serve as a means to feeling good. Makeup is my specialty, so I promote its value, but I respect anything that makes women appreciate themselves more. I have the good fortune to reach millions of television viewers who respond by letter and telephone. After hearing my message and trying new makeup techniques, my clients are thrilled with the results. The comments from them are so reassuring: "You know, you were right. I really feel better, and now I have a certain amount of confidence that I didn't have before." This is the kind of message they relay to me. In actuality, all that makeup has done is enhance exactly what is there to begin with, but the confidence of knowing they look their best changes their outlook.

Projecting one's own natural beauty is empowering. Without doubt, makeup is the most accessible and most effective tool for the least investment. It's also something we can use every day on our own at any time to create that confident feeling of being the best we can be.

Redefining Beauty

Mona Lisa wouldn't win any beauty contests, nor would we see her in the pages of fashion magazines—no high cheekbones, her lips aren't full, her eyes are on the small side. Da Vinci's lady meets none of the artificial standards of perfection that currently equate with beauty, yet her face has mesmerized the world for centuries. Given that she is completely dependent on the totality of her face, her special allure is absolutely unique. And, when other painters try to re-create her, it never works. Nor do the copies have any intrinsic value. Mona Lisa is one of a kind. And so is each of us.

For the last several decades, women, for whatever reasons, have been denying their unique good looks, preferring to copy the image of a select few beautiful women. In the 1940s they wanted to look like Rita Hayworth and Betty

Grable, 10 years later like Marilyn Monroe and Elizabeth Taylor, later like Audrey Hepburn and Natalie Wood. As models became the benchmarks of allure, the faces of Lauren Hutton, Cheryl Tiegs, Christie Brinkley, Brooke Shields, and Claudia Schiffer established more impossible standards. None of them set out to become paragons of perfection, yet suddenly women all over the world were trying desperately to look like them instead of themselves. But most of the time, as when the painters tried to duplicate the Mona Lisa, the clones didn't work. And the wannabes felt like failures.

As we approach a new century, redefining "beauty" is a must. To completely liberate women from the pressure to conform, we must first distinguish between a fashion fad and real beauty. Once that pressure is lifted, experimenting with fads can be fun again. This means that if a woman wants to follow a current vogue for very thin or full eyebrows, she can pluck or not pluck without feeling that her natural shape is somehow wrong. Or if the style is pale lips and dark eyes, she can test new makeups to give the look a try.

But if the "trend" is for very full lips or an upturned nose, she'll appreciate her own features enough that she won't rush off to a cosmetic surgeon for a permanent fix. When fashion dictates facial features, something's dreadfully wrong.

Beauty has a timeless quality. What's beautiful today is beautiful tomorrow. Fashion, on the other hand, is generally determined by fads. Fads are interesting, fun, and generate sales. Trends don't create beauty. What's stylish today is dated tomorrow. Any definition of beauty that includes a transitory quality is inaccurate and confusing.

A new definition of beauty can have no decrees of acceptability built into it. Women are too independent to accept such dictates. We cannot, as some researchers have actually done, attempt to calibrate specific standards that represent the "perfect" face. In one study a psychologist asked 150 white, male college-age men to rate the beauty of 50 women based on pictures of their faces. Only 13 of the women were non-white. From those responses the researcher calibrated the size and proportion of various features to come up with a numerical description of the "ideal" face. After reading the results of such a study, some desperate women will stand before a mirror, rulers in hand, trying to determine whether or not their mouths are half the width of their faces, their eye width is three-tenths the width, and the chin length one-fifth the length. Such inane specificity narrows an already limited general perception of what it really means to be beautiful.

No, a new definition of beauty must be much broader. By its guidelines all women should feel included rather than excluded. We should be able to look at ourselves realistically and appreciate what we see, not deprecate the reflection in the mirror because it doesn't meet a certain standard. By the new definition, beauty should be a positive in our lives, something that keeps us sane, not drives us crazy.

By expanding our concept of what is beautiful, we make room for all ethnic and racial groups. Rather than recognizing beauty by particular parameters, we should be looking at all different types and recognizing the loveliness that exists within each group. No group should be measured against the standards of any other—that would be too limiting. In the best of all worlds, we would limit the size of the groups to one individual and everyone would be recognized as beautiful; there would be no comparisons.

Okay, it is an imperfect world. We make comparisons. But the more different types we accept as beautiful, the more opportunity each of us has to feel good about our own particular style. Instead of clinging to old stereotypes, we can broaden our minds and see the glory in all kinds of faces. As more new icons of beauty are established, more of us are validated. Jaclyn Smith and Catherine Deneuve are still beautiful, so are Claudia and Brooke and Christie, and so, now, are Hillary Clinton, Oprah Winfrey, Barbra Streisand, and each of the distinctly different women you'll see in this book. There's no one way to be gorgeous anymore—the standards of beauty cross all lines.

To be meaningful, the true interpretation of good looks has to include more than just physical attributes. Self-confidence shows. Accomplishment shows. Kindness shows. The actress Jacqueline

Bisset once put it this way: "Character contributes to beauty. It fortifies a woman as her youth fades. A mode of conduct, a standard of courage, discipline, fortitude, and integrity can do a great deal to make a woman beautiful."

Now is the perfect time to put aside all the traditional and irrelevant standards of the past. We women have been moving in this direction for the last several years. We've grown more independent and more self-confident as we've recognized our own successes. I've observed the media gradually favoring and featuring new images of beauty. Advertising, editorial pages in magazines, films, and even television sitcoms are beginning to highlight diverse faces and body shapes that don't fit the old-fashioned stereotypes of beauty. That's because real women are speaking up, expressing their need to be accepted in all ways, including the way they look.

The new beauty is real, honest beauty. It's the whole spectrum of the way women look, feel, think, and act. All of these aspects have to be considered, because together they create the total image. Beauty can no longer be measured by male fantasies, Barbie dolls, and advertisements that try to force us into something we are not. Beauty is what each of us is born with. On a purely physical level, beauty is our reflection in the mirror. On a deeper level, it is our ability to accept that reflection.

When we open up the doors to the club that was once limited only to old-think "beauties," we eliminate the repressive aspect of attractiveness. If we redefine beauty to include all types of women, each of us has unlimited potential. We can feel good about our looks, enhance them any way we choose, and have fun with them. We'll be more accepting of our natural beauty. And we can finally concentrate on what's important, not what's in the mirror.

PART

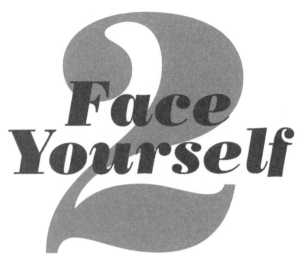

Face Yourself

Discovery is always exciting. When that discovery is your own beauty, it's a morale and confidence builder. When we stop comparing and actually give ourselves credit for being thoroughly beautiful individuals, we empower ourselves. That's when we have the confidence to act on our ideas and make our marks in the world. And that's when others recognize us as strong, competent and, yes, beautiful people.

Recognizing Your Essence in the Mirror

Before starting my cosmetics company, I spent 13 years as a makeup artist. During that time I worked on thousands of women's faces, and I can honestly say that I've observed the beauty in all of them. Since founding the company 5 years ago, I haven't met most of the women who wear my cosmetics, but I've read enough letters and spoken by phone with them often enough to know that they too are extremely special women. The essence of their beauty comes across whether I see them or not.

Very few women appreciate their own loveliness. When I was a makeup artist, it was often a huge challenge to work with clients, not because of their physical features, but because they were convinced that there was nothing attractive about their faces. Many women have spent most of their lives focusing on inadequacy. Never pretty enough. Too pale. Too dark. Too straight. Too crooked. Too big. Too small. Too fat. Too short. Too tall. You'd be amazed—or maybe you wouldn't be—how many women have never been told they are beautiful. These people have never felt attractive, and even if they are told that they look good, they don't hear it or they don't believe it. Instead they compare themselves to the media icons hyped as symbols of perfect beauty. Convinced that without oval faces, almond eyes, and thin, straight noses, they aren't pretty, they miss the special qualities of their own faces, their unique features that speak of diverse beauty.

Instead of celebrating their individuality, these women have spent billions of dollars trying to achieve cosmetic-ad perfection. In the quest to transform themselves into what I see as cookie-cutter blandness, they've hidden the very elements of their own allure. They hide their appealing eyes under too much eye shadow. They stripe their soft round cheeks with brown powders to feign gaunt-looking hollows. They coat their healthy complexions with thick foundations that could never be mistaken for natural.

I constantly urge women to get rid of all that! Makeup that's obvious…makeup that camouflages honest beauty. I tell them, "Wash it off and let the real you show." Once again, understand that I'm not urging anyone to throw out her makeup. Instead, I'm telling you, my readers, to use cosmetics as a grooming tool to enhance what you have, not to change a thing. I'm reminding you that no products will transform your face convincingly into someone else's.

I'm also suggesting that cosmetics that look as natural as possible will liberate you. My "no-make-up" makeup plan is one way of taking control of something tangible, something no one else owns—your face. You can make the most of your God-given beauty and simultaneously gain some self-confidence. When you realize, truly realize, how appealing your natural features are, you will feel comfortable with or without the extra cosmetics, and that's a definite ego booster.

Since you bought this book, I know you're willing to do a few simple exercises before experimenting with cosmetics. Here's the first one:

EXERCISE: Bend over from the waist, touch your knees, calves, or toes. Now just hang there for a moment and let the blood rush to your face. (You can do this seated on a chair, too, if standing is difficult—put your head between your knees.) Swing your body up and look at your refreshed image in a mirror. Brush your hair back so you can see yourself fully. Look at your face. First focus on each part: your hairline, forehead, brows, temples, eyes, eyelashes, nose, cheekbones, cheeks, lips, teeth, jawline, chin, complexion. Don't dwell on anything that you have considered to be a negative in the past. Instead look at the unique quality of each of your features. Next, concentrate on your entire face—the whole picture, the sum of those parts. Now write a list of at least 5 of the positive aspects about your face. If you can easily come up with 5, shoot for 10. If you can't come up with any, you're thinking too negatively. Ask your best friend for help—he or she will see them immediately. (Save the list, you'll be able to use it later when you analyze how to apply the most natural-looking makeup.)

Appreciating each feature, without comparing it with anyone else's, is a first step to recognizing your individual beauty. Each of those features is unique and—dare I say it again?—beautiful. The combination of them all is your face.

Few of us take the time to look at ourselves intently and focus on the positive. I've watched novice makeup artists working with women, pushing their faces all around, and I've heard them start listing all the "flaws," all the features to "adjust" and "erase." I see the women sinking lower and lower onto their chairs. No woman should hear a laundry list of what's "wrong" with her face—how degrading! When I analyze a woman's face I present the positives because that's what I see. Basically there are no "problems," short of inevitable acne breakouts or a scar that you hate, both of which can be helped easily with foundation. A face is a collage of features that is your personal statement.

5 Dispelling the Myths

Before we can accept our inherent natural beauty, we have to be willing to reject some of the faulty premises on which many of us, and centuries of women before us, have based our self-image. Together these archaic axioms create what has come to be known as "the beauty myth," because of a thought-provoking book of that title written in 1991 by Naomi Wolf. An ardent feminist, Wolf contends that the myth has undermined women by creating a "destructive obsession" that keeps us from achieving all that we can.

I'm convinced that certain unfounded assumptions about what is beautiful and what isn't impair our ability to accept our image. Once we erase these dictums from our collective conscience, accepting ourselves will be easier. And if all of us learn to appreciate ourselves and feel more self-confident, the pressure to conform to unrealistic guidelines will go away. It has to start with us.

Let's begin by getting rid of some misconceptions:

MYTH 1 *Looking younger means looking prettier.*

Prettier than what? How old does 40, 50, or 60 look? There has never been a better time in American history to disprove this myth. Since the "baby boomers" have reached their 40s and 50s, for the next few decades the population will be bulging with older people. The glamour of women over 40 will soon be fully appreciated (especially by those who have something to sell and recognize the buying power of 40+ women). Establishing 20-year-olds as the standard of beauty today is even more absurd than it has been in the past. The major difference now is that the majority of the population will soon reject the standard.

Never before have aging women had a loud, unified voice—their cries of "Enough, already!" haven't been heard. But now, because of their sheer numbers, those voices have developed into a powerful outcry. Television shows like "The Golden Girls" and magazines such as *Lear's* and *Mirabella* have already understood the message, and they're spreading it. The images they feature prove that aging faces can be beautiful, sensuous, and appealing; that gray hair is just another hair color; and that fashion exists to suit women of any age.

How many times have we heard that men get better with age, but women don't? I don't believe that at all. In the same way that men "grow into" their faces, so do women. Yes, certain aspects of anyone's face aren't as smooth and firm as they once were. But does a wrinkle look better on a man than a woman? I think not. There's a certain confidence and wisdom that shows on one's face and leaves a much deeper impression on others than age lines do. Most people find that aspect of aging very attractive.

By nixing the notion that we must look younger to look our best, perhaps women will feel less compelled to rush into plastic surgery. I shudder when I think of 30-year-old women going under the knife "to get rid of wrinkles" before they have any. These are the same women who end up having multiple surgeries before they reach 45, women whose faces have lost their personality. The faces don't look "younger," they look de-aged and artificial.

Don't misunderstand. Well-executed plastic surgery can make a woman look younger, and if having a procedure done makes her feel better and more confident, I would never discourage her. But I am cautioning against proceeding if she's feeling pressured into the operating room. Friends, lovers, career circumstances, and additional birthdays can create subtle anxieties that make women think they need to look younger to satisfy external demands. Such pressure is not a reason to subject oneself to serious surgery. Like makeup, exercise, and new clothes, plastic surgery can be a boon to self-esteem if it makes a woman feel more self-confident. But it's a very dangerous procedure if she believes it will dramatically change her life; her self-esteem may drop considerably when the surgery is over. Like any other superficial change, plastic surgery doesn't make things happen.

MYTH 2 *An oval face, small and straight nose, almond-shaped eyes, and full-lipped mouth are all "perfect" features.*

There's no such thing as perfect features. In fact, most of the time the most beautiful faces have distinctive features that are decidedly unlike the mythical description of perfection. Consider Lauren Bacall, Katharine Hepburn or Liza Minnelli; each has unique features that make their faces memorable. You'd recognize them with or without makeup. The models with so-called perfect faces often go unrecognized in a crowd.

As you will see in the how-to section starting on page 35, there is such a wide range of attractive features that referring to any single type as "perfect" is pointless. Yes, Candice Bergen has a beautiful nose and Jaclyn Smith's nose is exquisite. But equally gorgeous and distinctive are Barbra Streisand's, Meryl Streep's, and Sophia Loren's. That doesn't mean any of those noses are for everyone—they work on each unique face, not on every face. The point is to appreciate your own characteristics and enjoy your look as a sum of its parts, not fixate on any one feature.

MYTH 3 *It's essential to be thin.*

No, it's essential to be healthy. Obesity isn't healthy, but neither is starvation. What's most important is that you accept the reality of your body at every stage and not use it as reason to hate yourself or put off your own personal progress.

Surveys conducted by a number of different researchers have determined that 50 to 90 percent of women are unhappy with their bodies, especially their weight. However, based on statistics used by the insurance and medical industries, only 25 percent of females are overweight. That means that at least one-quarter of the 50 to 90 percent surveyed are upset about their bodies when they needn't be.

If you are carrying too much weight right now, you can do something about it. You have the power to help yourself achieve a healthy weight. When you are ready to start making changes in your life, you will—some people call it being in the "mood" to diet. Until you're ready for action, make peace with your body. Accept the fact that this is the body you have until you're ready to change it.

Enhancing a body—no matter what its shape—is what painters have done for centuries. To make the body look its very best, they play with light and shadow to create beautiful illusions. We're lucky that we can do that with makeup and hairstyles to flatter our faces and with clothing to complement the body. No—you won't look thin if you're currently overweight or round and curvaceous if you're underweight. But you will look the best for you right now. And you'll feel better about yourself than if you're hiding in shapeless camouflage garb or if you've given up on makeup and hair care.

Allowing the scale to determine when we buy new clothes, put on makeup, or get a haircut is a surefire way to sabotage high self-esteem. I've known women who've put off taking care of themselves "until I lose some weight," and they've ended up looking in the mirror and hating the reflection. Later on, in the chapter entitled "Role

Models," you'll read a real-life account of how one woman dealt with a similar situation.

MYTH 4 *Beauty equals success.*

It's easy to fall into the trap of believing this one. We read about gorgeous movie stars and models making millions of dollars; we see attractive news anchors interviewing some of the most famous people in the world; and we watch former beauty contest winners launch exciting careers. But that's the media influencing us. Many women's images wouldn't satisfy old artificial standards of beauty, yet each of their successes sets its own standards. Consider chef Julia Child, clothing designers Donna Karan and Liz Claiborne, Supreme Court Justice Sandra Day O'Connor, law professor Anita Hill, publisher Frances Lear, tennis ace Steffi Graf and ice-skater Kristi Yamaguchi. Not one of them is a classic beauty by the old definition, yet each is highly accomplished in her field.

Now think about their appearances. Isn't each of them lovely? Would we ever tire of looking at one of these women if she was reading the evening news? Not at all, because each is a believable beauty: credible, intelligent, and a major success. By a new, freer definition of beauty that incorporates a woman's actions and attitude as well as her healthy, unique appearance, each of these women should be on the cover of *Vogue*.

MYTH 5 *Beauty is in the eye of the beholder.*

You can't see me, but I'm shaking my head in total disagreement. Sometimes we hear things so many times that we lose sight of what these trite words actually mean. If we get romantically poetic about the statement, we can interpret it to mean that everyone has different tastes and that there are many interpretations of beauty. That's the most positive way of looking at that old saying. However, if we use the literal meaning, the sentence threatens our self-esteem. It gives away our individual power to define our own beauty and puts it in the hands of others, the beholders. When we know we are attractive, the world learns by osmosis. An upbeat attitude, a smile, and an image of obvious self-confidence comes across. We feel beautiful and look beautiful. When we let others become the judge of our image, we relinquish control, feel as though we need to meet or beat their standards to be acceptable, and quickly lose some of our confidence and self-esteem.

MYTH 6 Makeup will help you get a man/Men hate makeup.

I decided to deal with these together, since they address the same issue: relationships. How could makeup affect a relationship one way or the other?

For a moment, let's just forget the basic premise of my makeup system—that my makeup is so subtle that half the time nobody realizes you're wearing any, and if it is noticeable, it's not pronounced enough to cause comment. Although looking your very best may evoke a positive initial response from everyone you meet, makeup isn't going to make or break a relationship. In most surveys, men say that they notice a woman's eyes or her smile first. I believe that men are here

referring to the sincerity that comes across, not the specific feature. Both features can be enhanced with makeup, but the sincerity is all inside. Once two people start conversing, their personalities and individual levels of self-esteem come across, and the chemistry happens or it doesn't.

Now to the second part of this myth: Men hate makeup. Some do, some don't. Some like it very much. I say, who cares? If you like makeup, wear it. If you don't feel comfortable wearing it, don't. You know how you feel best. Don't be swayed by someone else's responses. If your relationship is going to work, the amount of makeup you wear isn't going to make an important difference.

MYTH 7 Elizabeth Taylor is the most beautiful woman in the world.

Once we start thinking that some women are more attractive than others, we fall into the beauty trap all over again. We get back into the habit of making unnecessary comparisons. Yes, Liz Taylor is beautiful in almost every photograph, film, and TV show we've ever seen. But is she more beautiful than you or anyone else? I doubt it.

When we let loose of those myths that for years have inhibited us from feeling good about ourselves and our choices, it's a great deal easier to shake some of the more explicit myths, the kind that are quicker to dispel: I call them the "makeup myths."

MAKEUP MYTH 1 *It takes a lot of money and time to look your best.*

Nobody knows better than I that it's easy to spend a great deal of money on makeup. Remember, I was once a makeup artist, and certainly no other group of consumers spends more on cosmetics (except perhaps for cosmetics executives, who are always on the lookout for what the competition is up to). But most women don't need to drop a fortune on beauty products.

As you'll see in the next section of the book, keeping makeup pared to the essentials is key to my natural makeup method. You don't need a vast array of colors, unless you want them, or expensive camouflage creams, highlight creams, contour powders, iridescent powders, or underbase preparations.

You don't need to shop in the most expensive places, either. There are fine quality products in drugstores and beauty supply shops. Although the color selection may be more limited (and even that's not always the case!), there is always a workable selection of shades.

In the section on foundation I provide you with tips for selecting the best foundation—that way you won't be buying base after base in search of the right shade. When you find the color and texture that works, stick with it. You'll also discover that once you have found the proper shade of foundation, you'll use far less since it's so easy to blend.

There are alternatives for saving time, too. Shopping from home or the office makes the most sense. Most of my clients never imagined that they'd be purchasing cosmetics by seeing them on television and ordering over the telephone. But now more than 1 million women order my products. Many others shop for their products via catalogs, and still others work with direct-sales representatives who come to their homes and workplaces.

MAKEUP MYTH 2 *Once you know your "season," you'll know exactly which cosmetic colors look best on you and which to avoid.*

I believe that every woman can wear any lipstick, blush, or eye makeup color that she wants to wear. It's ridiculous to tell a brunette that she can't wear purple or olive green or a redhead that she can't wear red. Limiting colors by overall eye and hair color is an outdated concept that is far too limiting. There's a shade of almost every color that flatters each individual. It takes some exploring to find them, but they are there. As I point out in the chapter on eye makeup, each individual has a multitude of colored flecks in her eyes, and I use these many colors as a key when selecting eye makeup.

The only two rules I follow are that the shades selected shouldn't be lighter than the complexion, and they should be coordinated (a brownish red lipstick with a berry blush and green eyeshadow doesn't work, but a deep pink lip, a medium pink blush, and pinkish brown eyeshadow does).

MAKEUP MYTH 3 *Everyone looks better with a tan.*

Back in the 1920s Coco Chanel decreed that a tan was chic, a sign of a class of people so moneyed that they could afford to loll in the sun for hours. That was before science determined that no tan is safe: extended exposure to ultraviolet light causes cumulative damage and can result in skin cancer. These days a tan is a symbol of disregard for our health—I wonder why anyone would want to look as if she has baked in the sun. That's why I don't suggest using fake-looking bronzing powders and artificial tanning creams and lotions. If you like a tan look, don't destroy your skin for the real thing—by all means use a self-tanning product. But rethink why you want darker skin—is it because of another old standard of beauty that needs to be reevaluated?

MAKEUP MYTH 4 *Makeup is all illusion.*

"Illusion" implies change, and as you know by now, I don't use cosmetics to change anyone's looks. I look at makeup as a tool that helps bring out the best in your face. Used properly, this tool does no magic, it doesn't alter anything; instead it enhances everything that's naturally beautiful about a face. The myth that makeup is all illusion developed back in the 1930s and 1940s when makeup was never subtle and phrases like "all dolled up" were used to describe a woman who was in full makeup and dress. The days of obvious makeup have been over since Joan Collins starred as Alexis Carrington in the last "Dynasty" episode.

The only time illusion figures into my makeup scheme is if someone is trying to camouflage a temporary problem or do minor corrective makeup on a particular feature that bothers her. Then shadow and highlight can create some illusions, but in that case they serve a purpose.

MAKEUP MYTH 5 *Some women can wear the "natural" look and others just can't.*

Everyone can enhance their own natural beauty with a minimum of makeup. There's nothing more natural than that, short of not wearing any at all. My friend actress Lisa Hartman told me that she was one of those people who thought she had to wear layers of makeup to look her best. This was how Lisa explained the story of her transition: "I got caught up in the trends. At one time it was very 'in' to wear a ton of makeup, and I did. But one day I looked in the mirror and also saw some pictures of myself. I realized that I was heavily made up—I had crossed the line of good taste, especially with eye makeup. But wearing too much makeup had become a habit with me. It was difficult to go back to a look of purity and simplicity. But each day I started wearing less and less. Now there are many days when I don't wear anything at all, and I feel perfectly comfortable. For me, the whole concept of 'less is more' makes perfect sense. I actually feel prettier now than I did then. Part of that comes from being more comfortable with myself, too, in my thirties."

Getting Started

I spend most of my working hours developing products that help women look their best. But, quite honestly, good products and makeup techniques are only part of looking great. Mental attitude is another. The third integral component is physical. What we eat and our exercise, sleep patterns, and grooming routine are essential to a glowing, healthy appearance. Many doctors use the skin as a gauge of overall health. They check its color, texture, temperature, sensitivity, and moisture levels when assessing various medical problems. Even psychiatrists get indications of anxiety, depression, and stress by observing the skin, the largest organ in the body. Fortunately this is the one organ that is constantly revitalized, cells shedding and regenerating in a 30-day cycle. A healthy body is reflected by its healthy outer covering.

The skin is basic to our bodily functions—it helps us breathe, sense, ventilate, excrete, defend against disease, regulate body temperature, store nutrients, and protect against shock and the elements. But there's form in all that function—our epidermis is attractive, too. Nothing is quite as beautiful as a clear, glowing skin.

Of course, everyone would like to have the complexion they were born with: beautiful, baby-soft skin. As soon as the umbilical cord is cut, however, the skin starts aging. By the time each of us hits our teens, twenties, and beyond, our skin has aged accordingly. Sun, pollution, stress, and inconsistent diet and exercise habits can add up to troubled skin. Some problems are genetic or hormonal, like acne, and we can't control them, but in most cases we can take positive actions to defend our skin as well as it defends us.

I've developed some simple systems for myself that work for my schedule. I've shared my ideas with friends; they've tried them and had good results. Since everything I do to care for myself is based on the most natural methods, I hope some of my ideas will help you. My approach has always been K.I.S.S. (Keep It Simple, Sweetheart!). By following a few easy suggestions that you can adapt to your life-styles, you'll find ways to keep your skin looking fantastic.

Nutrition

Nurturing our bodies with healthy food and plenty of water is the fastest way I know to glowing good looks. Most nutritionists will recommend that clients drink 6 to 8 glasses of water each day. Once in this habit, water drinkers comment that their skin shows immediate benefits: blemishes diminish, fine lines are minimized, and the skin looks refreshed. A balance of fruits, vegetables, and complex carbohydrates such as breads, pastas, and rice provide most of the nutrients our cells need to flourish. Add to these essential food groups moderate to low amounts of protein, dairy, and fat for complete nourishment and energy.

Erratic dietary habits wreak havoc on our system, and our skin shows the inner chaos almost immediately. People who are always on diets usually complain that their skin breaks out intermittently or gets dry and laced with fine lines. The body is trying to stabilize in reaction to the unpredictable nourishment it is receiving. The breakouts are a temporary condition that actually indicates something positive is going on: the body is cleaning out toxins. If the condition persists, however, it's best to see a dermatologist. Dryness may be a response to a low-fat diet. Since many of us are trying to lower the fat content in our diets, we should be aware that the outermost layers of the skin may suffer. Fine lines on the face and a crepey appearance on the hands and feet often occur when dietary fat content falls below 15 percent. Should that happen, increase the amount of water you drink and apply adequate moisturizer to keep the skin lubricated.

Exercise and Relaxation

I admit it. I hate "exercise programs." You know the kind. An hour of weights 2 or 3 times a week and 4 or 5 days a week of planned aerobics. I immediately feel guilty if I miss a few days, and when I'm doing it, I watch the clock, anxious for the program to be over.

Maybe you're one of the lucky people who enjoys that method of exercise. If so, know that I used to aspire to be like you. I tried every different exercise class and weight workout I could find. There was nothing I could stick to. But I've grown to accept myself and my preferences. I now know it's okay not to follow a prescribed plan.

I also know that it's not okay not to exercise my body, for health reasons primarily and for aesthetic reasons, too.

To stay physically fit and relatively trim, I've learned to make some choices that include an aerobic workout as often as I can. I make a concerted effort to have fun while I move. I walk, long walks when possible, short walks if that's all the time I can allot. I play tennis, racquetball, and basketball, and I swim and ride horses whenever I can. If my son, Evan, wants me to go outside for a game of catch and I want to read a book, I play catch. If I have an appointment on a second- or third-floor office, I challenge myself to take the stairs. Sometimes I'll even do four flights, for the fun of it. No matter what, I do something active that gets extra oxygen flowing into my system every day.

Now I never resent exercise because I make movement choices that are fun for me, choices that can't help but improve my physical condition. I've learned from exercise specialists and doctors that a brisk 20-minute walk 4 times a week will keep me in a healthy state, and anything more than that will improve my condition. I said good-bye to exercise guilt.

The other big plus about exercise is that it helps keep skin clear. As the circulation improves and the body works up a sweat, impurities are flushed out of the system. I love how my face looks after a quick walk into town or a fast game of tennis. Those are the times I'm happy to just wash my face and forget about wearing any makeup.

As important as exercise are sleep and relaxation. We've all got too much to do, too much to think about, and too much pressure. We have to give ourselves time to rest. I try to sleep at least 8 hours every night. If I can sleep 10 hours on a weekend, I relish the luxury. Usually, though, I'm lucky to get a full 8 hours. I find that if I take short breaks during the day to leave my office and sit on a different chair, or lie down on a sofa for 5 or 10 minutes, I feel refreshed. Sometimes, with my schedule, I can't afford the luxury, so I just relax at my desk with my eyes closed and do some deep-breathing exercises. Try the one above.

> **EXERCISE:** Sit on the edge of your chair with your feet planted firmly on the floor, back straight, hands relaxed on each thigh. Eyes closed. Slowly and smoothly inhale through the nose to the count of 5. Exhale very slowly through the mouth to the count of 5. As you exhale, make a concerted effort to roll and relax your shoulders. Make sure your spine is straight. Repeat 3 times. Eventually repeat 5 or 6 times.

Preparing Your Skin for "No-Makeup Makeup"

In the same way that I can't do a complex exercise program every day, I'm not one who devotes 45 minutes to facial cleansing every morning and night. I simply don't have time. Instead I have simplified my routine to suit my life.

Here's my basic morning routine:

I wash my face with my gentle cleanser, which dissolves the excess oils and kills the bacteria that accumulate overnight. I don't use soap now because it's too drying, but when I was younger I used only soap. You have to experiment and see what works best for you. After you cleanse, your face should not feel taut and dry on the surface. If it does, the product is too drying.

Next I use a toner. Mine is a spray that contains collagen, elastin, and aloe vera, to stimulate the skin, refine the pores, and get rid of minute traces of cleanser. Be certain that whichever toner you choose is alcohol free.

My final step is to apply a light moisturizer. If I'm going to be out in the sun, I use sunscreen all over my body except my face, and I reapply it often. Because, like many women, my face is very sensitive, I break out when I apply sun products to my face. That's a problem. But I make sure that I wear a foundation that has a sunscreen built into it, and I wear a hat with a deep brim. If it's an especially bright day, I try to stay out of the sun between 11 A.M. and 2 P.M., when the rays are the most dangerous.

At night the routine is almost the same:

Since my cleanser is a dual-action product—a makeup remover and facial wash in one—I eliminate one step. (If you use traditional products, dissolve your makeup first with makeup remover, then cleanse.) I follow with toner, eye gel, and moisturizer. At least twice a week I treat myself to a masque to deep-cleanse the pores, tighten them and rid the surface of the skin of any accumulated dead cells.

If my routine was more complicated, I probably wouldn't stick to it. Except for the nights when I use a masque, I'm ready for bed in about 3 minutes. That's the way I like it.

Now, about Your Makeup

In the next 96 pages you'll learn how to enhance everything that's beautiful about you. Remember when I asked you to make a list of your best features? Go back to that list and keep it handy. If you have great eyes, concentrate on the eye chapter. If lips are your best asset, follow the steps for playing them up.

In the beginning of the makeup section I show you how little time it takes to achieve a very natural look: 2, 5, or 10 minutes. Suit yourself. Only you know how much time you can afford. Maybe there are days or evenings when you want to spend more time—if so, enjoy the process and relish the results. The first few times you try my techniques, it may take you a bit longer, but with some practice you'll master all the quick-and-natural makeup techniques. Experiment and enjoy the process!

The No-Makeup Look

My goal is to make every woman look and feel her best. For some that means little or no makeup, for others it's a more glamorous attitude with dramatic lips and eyes. Once you master my "no-makeup" methods, you can minimize or intensify colors to suit your mood and personal style. The point is to appreciate your face with or without makeup.

Makeup in 2, 5, and 10 Minutes

SIBEL
After

After 2 minutes

The 2-minute makeup is the ultimate "less is more" statement. I use this minimalist approach most of the time in my own life—it's convenient, efficient, and effective. In 120 seconds I put on my foundation, highlight my eyes and cheeks, play up my lips a bit, and I'm out the door. As a working mom, I have little time to devote to my face, so I use the same quick, easy routine most mornings.

In Sibel's case, a light makeup accents her bone structure and her dark eyes, both of which can look very dramatic on the days and nights she decides to use more makeup (see those results on the next two pages). She applies foundation sheerly all over her face, including on her eyelids. The base smooths out the shadows around her nose and chin. When she has blended it all completely, she uses a clean sponge to blend again and absorb any excess. The whole foundation process takes about 45 seconds. A few strokes of brow pencil strengthens Sibel's brows—5 seconds each brow. In 5 seconds she adds a light touch of eye shadow—most of discoloration on her lids is covered with the foundation. She lines her top and bottom lids with taupe pencil and smudges the line to a soft shadow—10 seconds each eye. She wears one coat of mascara, top and bottom—5 seconds each eye. She dusts her cheekbones with peach blush—5 seconds each cheek. For lasting lip color, Sibel lines and colors her lips with peach pencil—20 seconds.

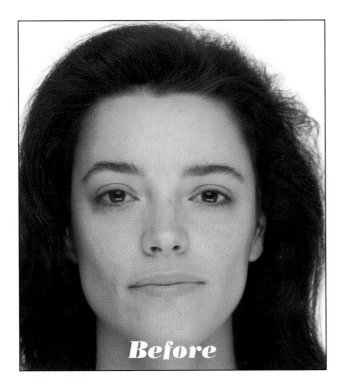

Before

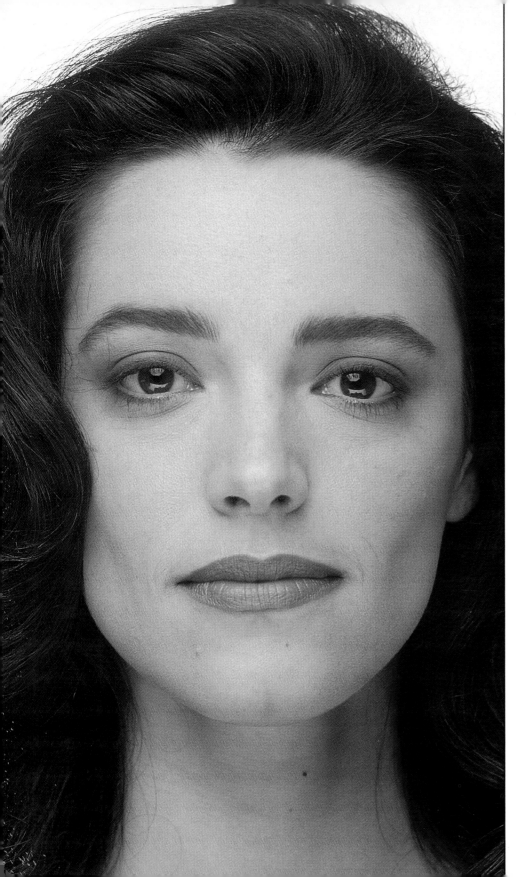

After 5 minutes

Special meetings and social occasions sometimes call for more complete make-up. Sibel spends the extra time defining her eyes. She intensifies the eyeliner a bit on each eye. However, adding the liner and eye shadows—as many as three well-blended colors—won't take more than two minutes. To intensify the cheek color after the eyes are complete, takes another 10 seconds for each cheek. The remaining 40 seconds can be devoted to lipstick, especially if she blends her own shade. With a little practice it takes far less time.

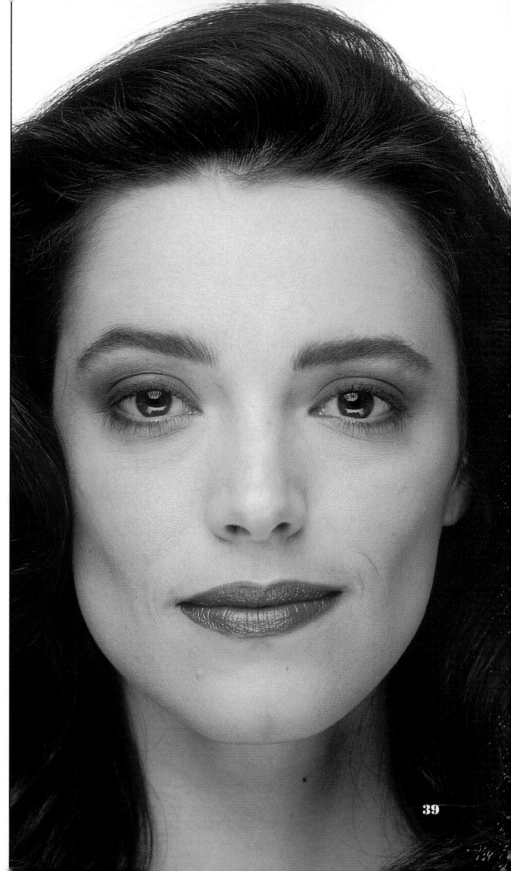

After 10minutes

Sibel has an angular face that can look very sophisticated, particularly if she uses two shades of blush to emphasize the chiseled look of her cheeks. Blending the cheeks carefully to avoid a war-paint look takes extra time. Allow 90 seconds per cheek. In addition, Sibel's brows are darkened a bit more, her eye shadows have been intensified, and her lips are lined with red and colored with red lipstick—2 extra minutes. The results: the 10-minute face. Sibel uses this look for special occasions only.

ELIZABETH

After

After 5 minutes

Ask most women how long they spend with their makeup and they'll tell you "5 minutes max." In that amount of time, you can achieve some wonderful effects with makeup. When I'm getting ready for business meetings or going out for dinner, I spend the extra few minutes on makeup that it takes to make me feel special. I pay more attention to my eyes, adding more shadows and

mascara, yet I try never to lose the natural look. I don't want to look dramatically different than I normally do, but I also want other people to concentrate on my eyes, so the extra effort and time is worth it.

Look at the tremendous difference those few minutes make in Elizabeth's looks. By devoting a full minute or minute and a half to applying her foundation, she is able to minimize the shadows under her eyes and around her nose and mouth. Her beautiful dark eyes and nicely shaped brows come to life with a few shades of shadows, pencil, and mascara. Her brows take about 15 seconds each, and her liner, shadows and mascara require about 60 seconds each. Blush on both cheeks takes a total of 30 seconds, and lining and coloring her lips consumes another 30.

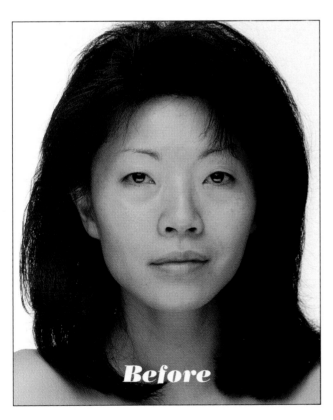

Before

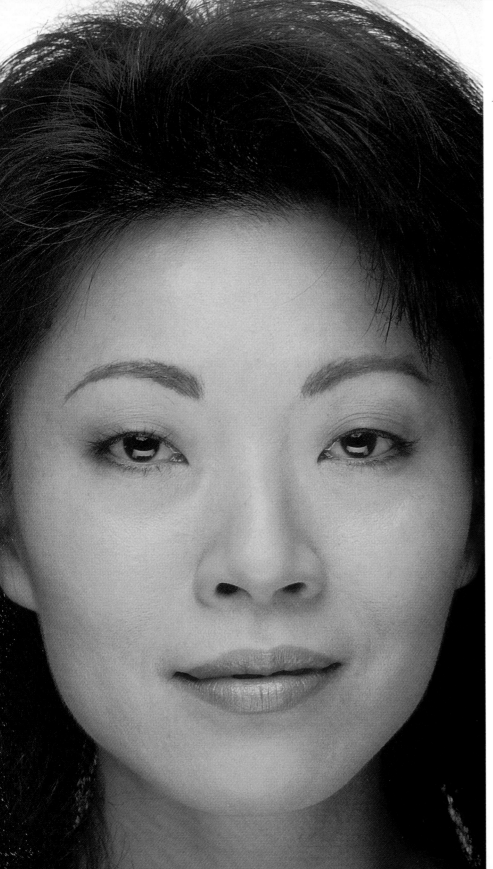

After
2 minutes

When Elizabeth has limited time, she can spend most of it on her eyes. It takes about 30 seconds to apply and blend foundation only on the parts of the face that need it most—under the eyes and around the nose. Add 10 seconds for pencil on each brow, 25 seconds to shadow, line, and add mascara to each eye. No more than 5 seconds for a hint of blush. The final touch—fifteen seconds for lip pencil to line and color lips.

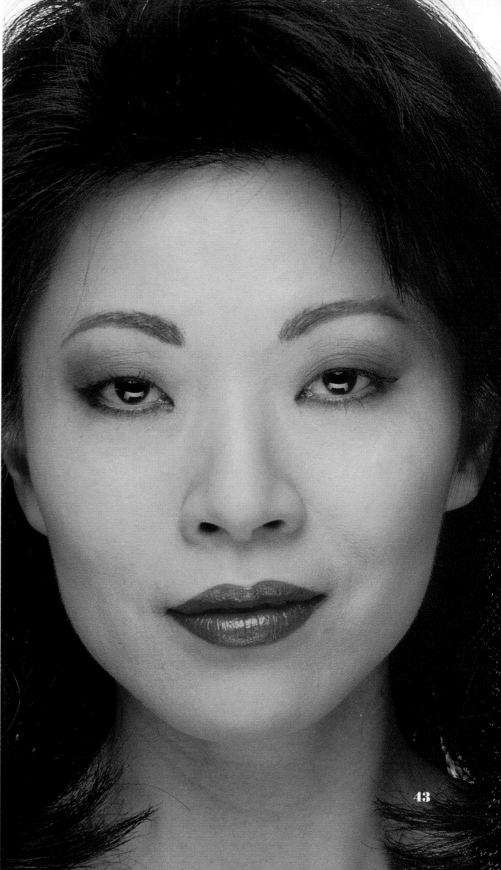

After 10 minutes

Ten minutes allows for the addition of liquid eyeliner, which takes about 15 seconds per eye but adds definition that immediately makes the eye look bigger. Blending three shades of shadow to add some depth to her lid area takes another 60 seconds for each eye. Allow about 10 seconds for lower liner. Two coats of mascara on each eye takes about 40 seconds. Shadowing her nose bridge to give the nose a slimmer look takes about 90 seconds. Except that she uses deeper shades of blush and lipstick, the time required is still just a minute altogether. She's done in about 8 minutes.

43

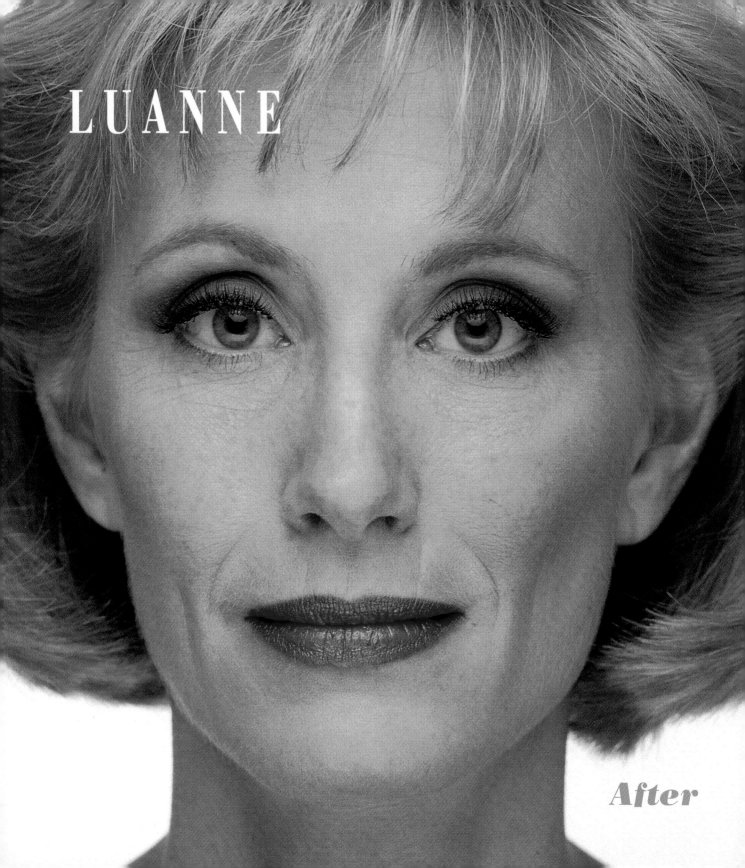

LUANNE

After

After 10 minutes

Spending 10 minutes on makeup doesn't necessarily mean that you're getting ready for a special occasion—it could be your daily operating procedure. (I know some women who spend 20 minutes, and I wonder what they can do for so long—but that's okay, they obviously enjoy the process!) Some women are very precise about every application and place a high priority on how their makeup looks. Others spend 10 minutes getting ready for a television appearance. Your individual priorities determine how much time you spend.

As you'll see on these three pages, Luanne looks wonderful no matter how much makeup she wears. This 10-minute procedure provides a very glamorous image, yet she doesn't look like she's wearing much. The key is perfectly applied foundation that's sheer and well blended. Even a complicated foundation application that involves two shades for subtle contouring won't take more than 2 1/2 minutes at the most. Adding definition to the eyebrows with a soft pencil adds about 45 seconds per brow. Well-defined eyes blended with three or four shadows, liner, and several coats of mascara require about 3 minutes total. After some practice most women can even apply a pair of false eyelashes in only 2 minutes. Blush takes 30 seconds, and lips can be lined and colored with lipstick in 30. Ten minutes well spent (and without the lashes, it's done in 8!).

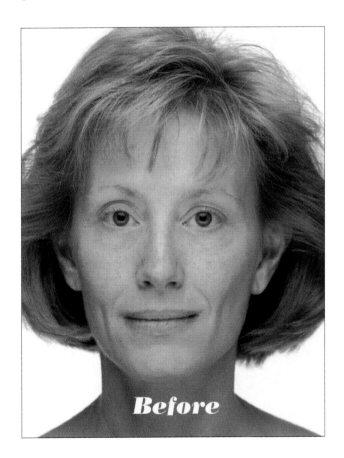

Before

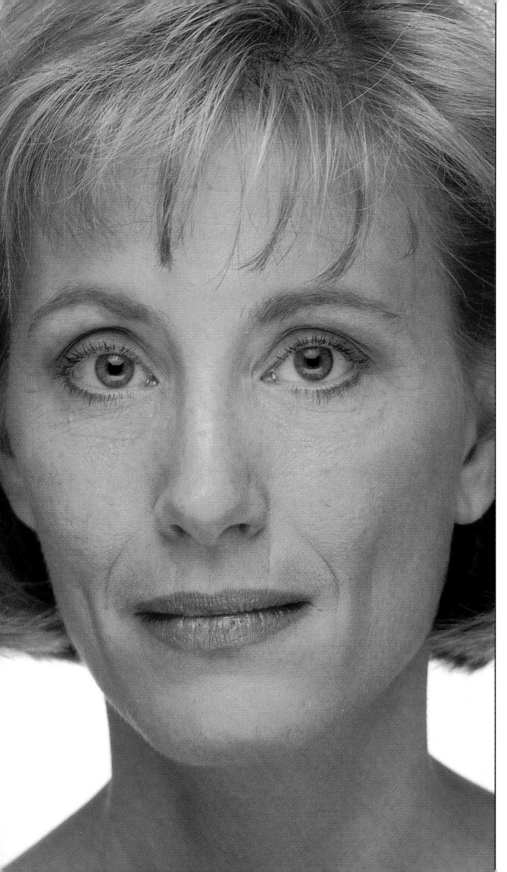

After
2 minutes

For a very clean and natural no-makeup look, Luanne's foundation takes about 40 seconds, blending carefully under the eyes. The eyes are lined, and the line is smudged in less than 20 seconds for both eyes. A light application of earth-tone shadows takes 10 seconds. Blush on cheeks takes a total of 15 seconds. Lips get a nice finish in 20 seconds—that's lined and filled in with pencil. Take another 10 seconds to add touches of blush on nose and chin, and there's still time to spare.

After 5 minutes

To take the 2-minute make-up to a less sporty stage, more eye makeup and blush make the difference. Blending three shades of neutral-toned shadow and intensifying the liner, especially on the outer corner of the lower lid, takes a minute more on each eye. Blush is used to add angles to the cheekbones, which requires only another 20 seconds. Brush-on lip color over the penciled lips is an additional 15 seconds. That's still less than 5 minutes for a finished look that works day or evening.

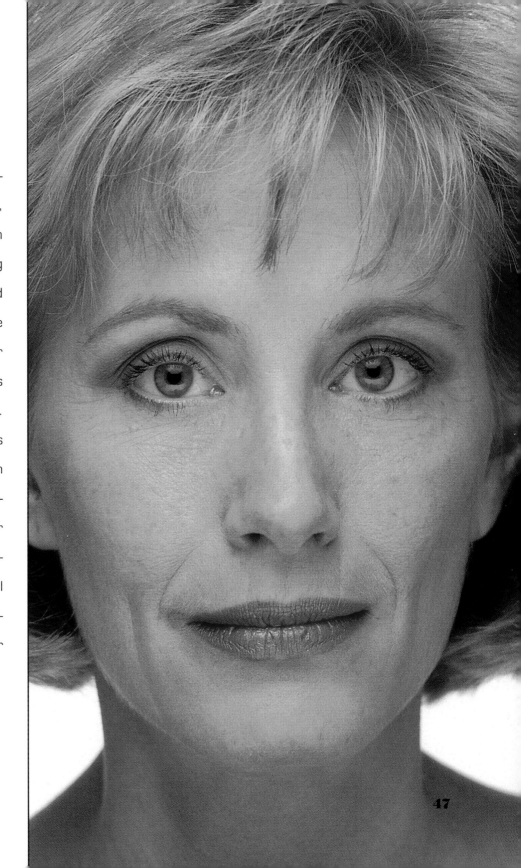

47

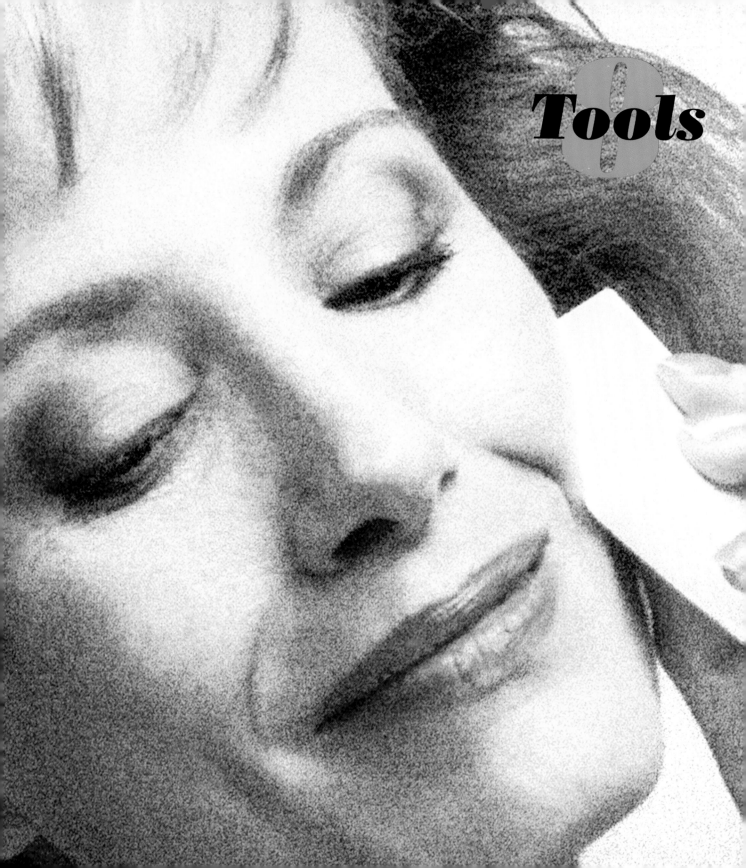

Tools

Professional results require professional tools. That's why I've spent so much time selecting the brushes and applicators that I use at home and those that come with my makeup. The implements that fit in compacts are limited by their size, however. Over the years I've found that a few full-size tools make the process easier, quicker, and more effective. I'll describe my favorites, then you decide what you need.

When I package my foundation in its compact, I include a rectangular sponge that's perfect for on-the-go applications and quick touch-ups. But when I'm at home, I use a latex wedge sponge. Its sharply defined edges make it easy to apply and smooth foundation in small crevices around the nose and under the lower lashes, and to clean up excess base that may accumulate in laugh lines.

Some women prefer a powder puff that is softer and thicker than those that fit in compacts. Personally, I prefer the compact style because a flat puff can conform to facial contours for exact placement. Try both and choose your favorite.

Four tools that I rely on for natural-looking eye makeup and brow grooming include tweezers (your brows should always be carefully groomed; see the brow chapter for more details), a brow brush that has a brush on one side and a comb on the other (to keep brows smooth and emphasize the shape), an eyelash curler (to make your lashes look their longest), and an eyelash-separating comb (to eliminate the clumps that can occur with mascara).

I designed a special eye shadow brush with bristles on both ends. It's great for applying and blending color on the lid. I use the full tip for blending. The other end has a slanted tip, which I shaped especially to apply shadow at an angle at the outer corners of the eyes. I've found that the dual eye shadow brush can be used for more than just eye makeup. Because the brushes are rather firm, I use the slanted end to achieve shading and highlighting effects that I describe

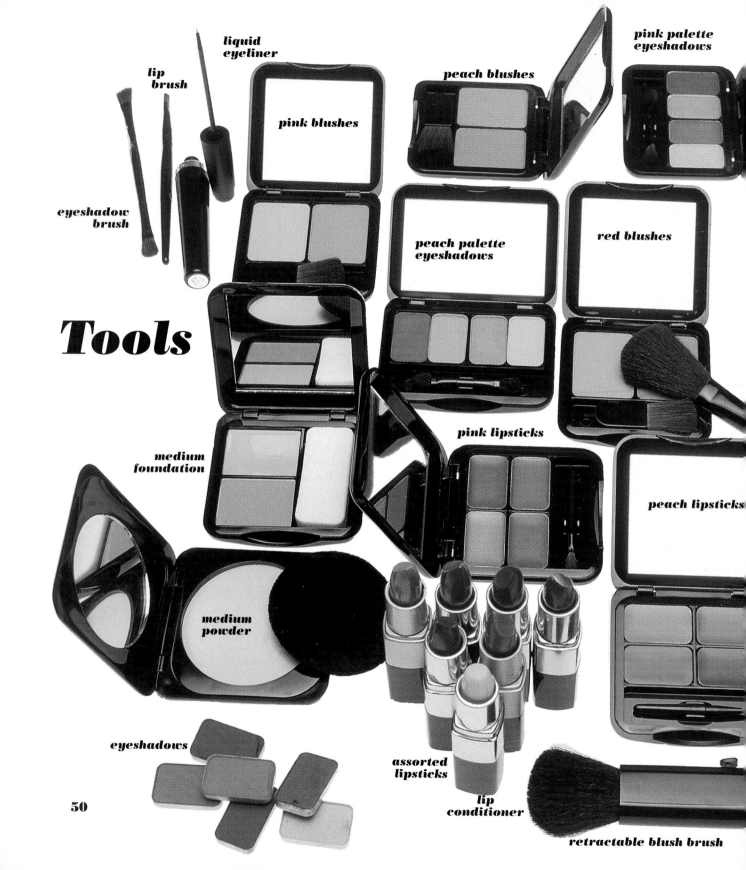

lip brush

liquid eyeliner

pink blushes

peach blushes

pink palette eyeshadows

eyeshadow brush

peach palette eyeshadows

red blushes

Tools

medium foundation

pink lipsticks

peach lipsticks

medium powder

eyeshadows

assorted lipsticks

lip conditioner

retractable blush brush

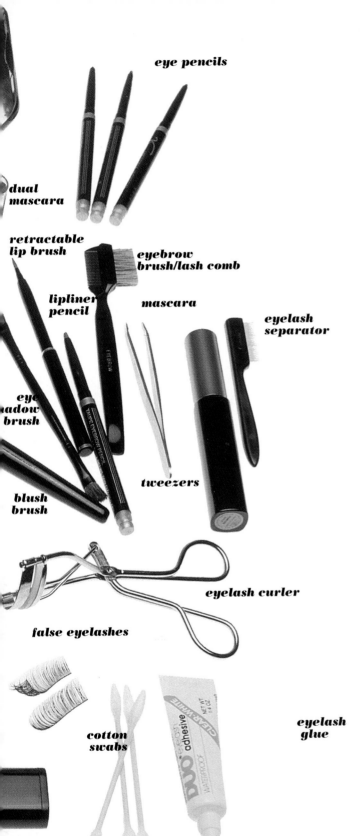

eye pencils

dual mascara

retractable lip brush

eyebrow brush/lash comb

lipliner pencil

mascara

eyelash separator

eye shadow brush

tweezers

blush brush

eyelash curler

false eyelashes

cotton swabs

eyelash glue

later in the "Unique Features" section. I often use the full tip to apply foundation to dark circles under the eyes.

Big fluffy brushes are best for blush application—choose one that's about one-half inch at its bristle base. Once you get used to using a blush brush with a long handle, the compact-size brush may no longer please you. In that case, try a retractable blush brush that's small enough for your purse yet still offers length and soft full bristles.

When I'm away from home, I always use the small applicator and brush that come in my lip color compact. But when at home, I use a longer brush for more control. If you get accustomed to the longer length, you can purchase retractable versions that are convenient for your purse. Remember, using a lipstick brush provides the most control and the most natural finish.

51

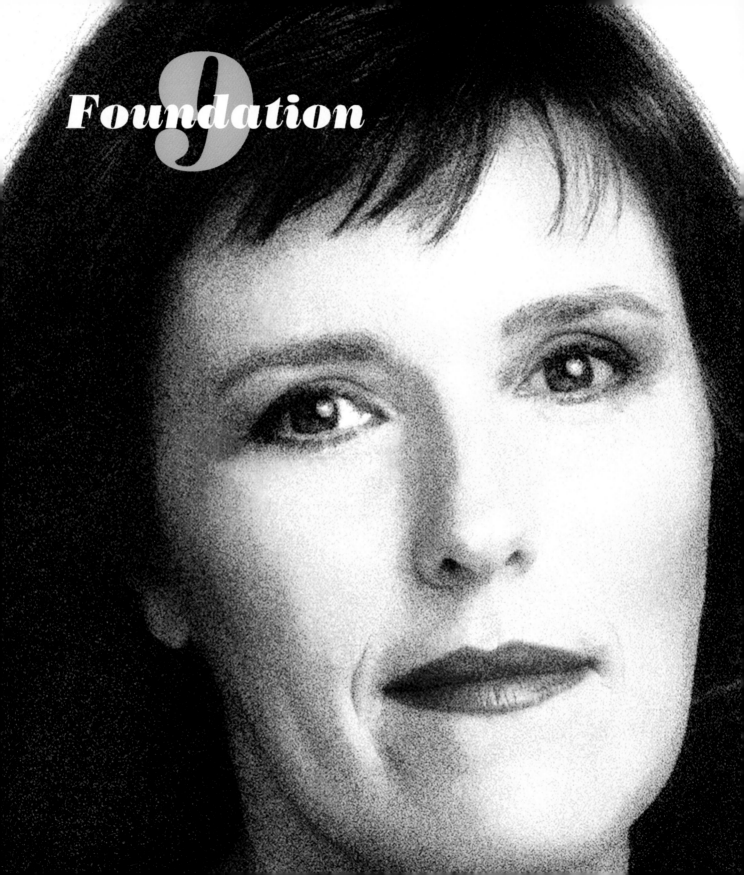

Foundation

Foundation is near and dear to my heart. After all, that's how I got my start in the cosmetics business. Finding the right color and texture of base had always been my biggest problem as a makeup artist. I wanted something that would be sheer and a cover-up—something that wouldn't hide the natural glow yet would conceal blemishes and uneven tones when necessary. I was also very aware that in both social and professional situations women always complained to me about their foundation—wrong color, wrong consistency, just plain wrong. Obviously, finding a good base wasn't only my problem—it's universal. That's why I decided to formulate my own product. Today it's my best-selling item!

The proper foundation will match your complexion exactly. When it's on, it will minimize the redness of broken capillaries, the dark circles under your eyes, and the splotchiness that can be caused by everything from acne and aging to a faded tan and pregnancy. And most important, the right base will allow you to show through.

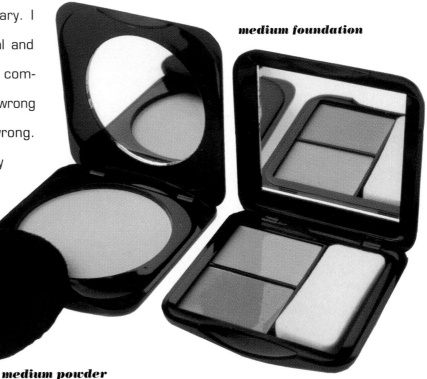

medium foundation

medium powder

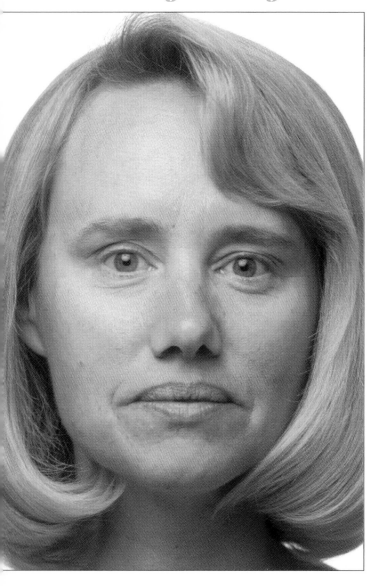

Elizabeth has quite a bit of redness in her complexion and discoloration around her nose and mouth. A foundation with a pink cast would exaggerate the redness.

I've seen many famous faces without foundation, and I'm here to tell you, nobody has "perfect" skin. If a star's complexion looks flawless, it's because she has found the perfect base. Like most women, celebrities are absolutely loyal to their favorite foundation. When they find the product that suits their complexion, they rarely ever change. That's why Ali and Meredith are so dedicated to my foundation—it works for them.

Strange as it may sound, selecting the right foundation is critical to the "no-makeup" look. It evens skin tones and refines the look of the complexion. Most women look fresher and more naturally beautiful wearing a bit of foundation, but many balk at the idea because they think base doesn't look natural.

They've been wearing the wrong product.

When you apply the foundation that's right for you, you look as if you're not wearing any at all. When you find *your* foundation, with the color and consistency that suits your complexion, don't stray from it. There's no need to. The color of your complexion shouldn't vary noticeably unless you are exposed to excessive sunlight (I certainly hope you're not determined to get a tan; exposure to ultraviolet light is directly related to skin cancer—and if that's not enough to scare you, remember that wrinkles are the result of cumulative sun damage). So once you find the right shade, it should suit your complexion for a long time. Although many makeup artists recommend having a summer and a winter shade, I find that in most cases the same foundation shade will suffice year round.

The proper shade will look invisible on your skin. To find your best shade, start by eliminating all the bases with a pink, gray, or orange undertone. If you can't visualize what I mean, it will become clear when you see the bottles and compacts lined up at the cosmetics counter. Choose a foundation that has a yellow or neutral undertone. That will help to cut any excess redness in your skin. If your complexion is sallow with a touch of green to it, a pink-based foundation will not balance it—instead it will make you look muddy and artificial. I'm convinced that a foundation with yel-

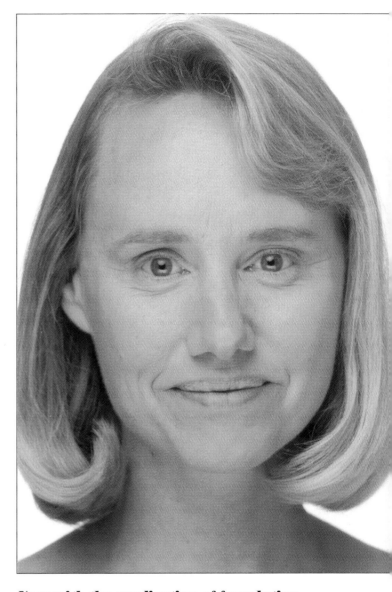

Now with the application of foundation and no other makeup, Elizabeth's skin tones are much more even. The correct base for her has a yellow undertone that cuts the redness. Notice how the minor discolorations have disappeared even without concealer.

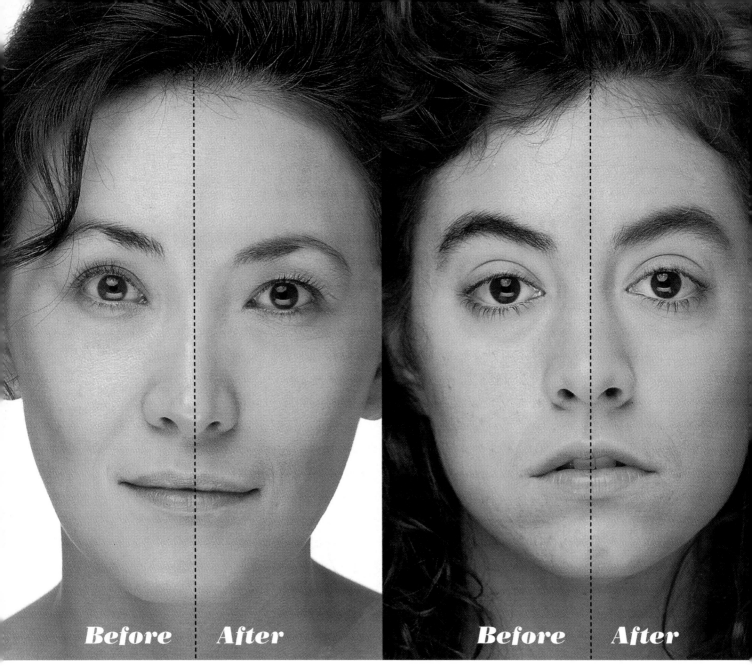

Before   **After**

Before   **After**

Kaoru, above, has flawless pale skin that can assume a greenish cast against her black hair. A light, neutral-beige foundation without any pink is most flattering. To keep her foundation sheer, she adds a touch of moisturizer to the sponge before applying foundation.

Andrea, above, has an olive complexion common to many women of Hispanic, Middle Eastern, and Mediterranean extraction. She has to be careful not to wear foundation with a pink, green, or gray tone. A medium beige suits her.

low or neutral undertones works on most women of all races. The few who have very pink skin may like the effect of counterbalancing the all-over flush with ivory foundation.

Always test shades on your jawbone until you find the one that exactly matches your face and neck. We've all seen women who look like they're wearing masks because their faces are a different color from their necks—surely those are the women who tested their base on their wrist, a spot that doesn't match either the face or the neck. Make sure that you have on no foundation when you test a new base—even a little will make a difference. Once you've blended the right shade on your jaw, you should not see a line of demarcation. It should blend into your skin, not sit in a thick layer on top of it. Your skin tone should look even and more refined. Don't be satisfied that you've selected the right shade by looking in a mirror inside a store or in your home. Step outside and check it in the daylight. (If you're shopping at night, ask for a sample and try it on at home the next morning.) By the way, if you do buy a new base and find when you get home that it's the wrong color, take it back immediately and exchange it for the proper shade! Cosmetics companies want you to find the right shade—we know you're loyal to the product that suits you best, especially a foundation shade.

Your foundation should be sheer. Even if you have spots to cover up, select a base that lets your own skin texture show through—that's part of your natural beauty. If you try to change anything dramatically, you will end up looking artificial. Later I'll show you how to minimize scars, small lines, and other problems that might bother you. But don't slather on a thick layer of makeup trying to cover them. There are better ways!

I'm a fan of cream makeup—obviously, since that's the only kind I make. I find that it's much easier to control the coverage. But if you get good results with a liquid, mousse, or cake form, by all means use what works for you. I've developed my foundation without any oil, so it achieves the matte finish of oil-free liquids yet still can be blended easily.

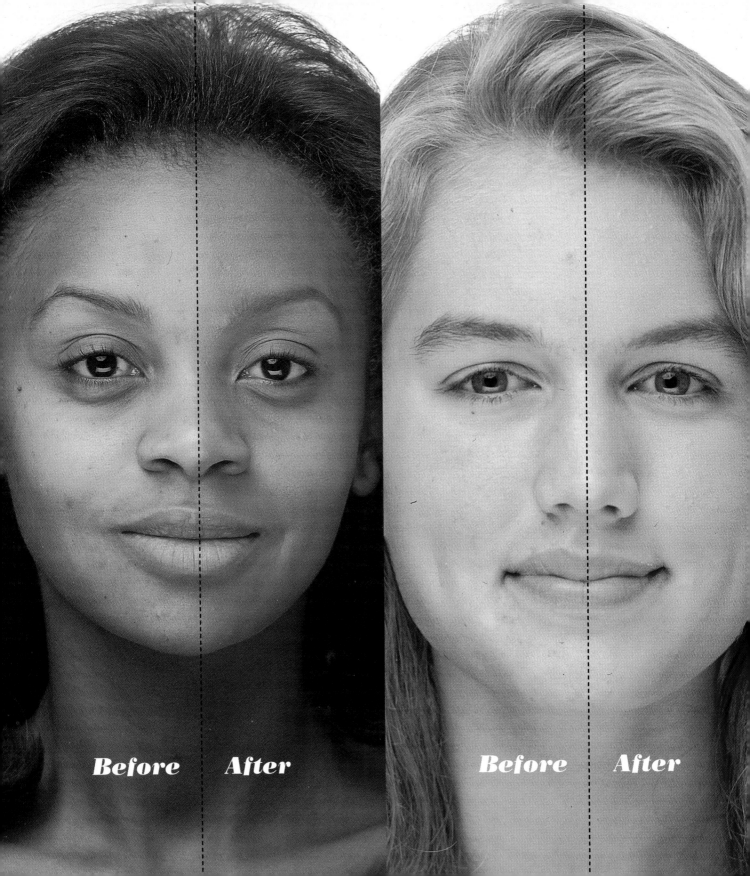

Before   **After**   **Before**   **After**

Should You Wear Foundation?

Yes, if it makes you feel prettier. If you look in the mirror and see an improvement, that's reason enough.

Yes, if you are comfortable wearing it.
Today's foundations are so lightweight that wearing one is a pleasure.

Yes, if it's sheer and lets your natural skin texture show through.
Less is always more when it comes to foundation.

Yes, if you fixate on minor skin imperfections. Broken blood vessels, shadows, and blemishes can be minimized with a sheer foundation.

Yes, if other people can't tell you're wearing it.
When you've selected the right color and texture, foundation is virtually invisible.

No, if you feel unnatural and self-conscious wearing base.
For some women, any makeup is too much.

No, if your skin is sensitive to or irritated by it.
Don't aggravate a problem.

No, if you lack the patience to blend carefully.
You won't like the finished result.

No, if your skin pleases you exactly the way it is!
The best reason of all to skip it!

Camey, opposite left, like many African-American women, has both red and green undertones in her dark skin. These are to be enhanced, not masked with ashy gray or orangy foundations. Here she uses her sponge to blend a mix of a dark reddish brown and a midtoned tan with a slightly golden undertone. Lisa, opposite right, has teenage skin with breakouts. After paying special attention to the breakouts (see page 63), she can still wear a sheer foundation that helps cut the surface redness in her complexion. To cover her blemishes, she applies medium foundation directly on the blemishes using a stippling technique, then blends with the sponge to create a smooth, sheer finish.

Tips for Selecting the Best Color

• Pick a shade as close as possible to your natural complexion color—don't try to alter your skin color with foundation.

• Always test foundation on your jawline. A perfect match means a stroke of the base on your jaw will be invisible.

• When testing a shade, your skin should be free of any other foundation.

• You may need to buy two foundations and blend them together to achieve a perfect match. Don't blend them in the bottles; blend shades with your applicator sponge.

• Make your final decision only when you see yourself in natural light. Indoor lighting can be misleading.

• Instead of using concealer on spots that need lightening, use a foundation one-half to one shade lighter than the shade you use on the rest of your face.

• If your skin gets darker in summer, select a foundation one-half to one shade darker than your regular shade. Use the regular shade as your summertime light.

I always package my foundations in pairs—a light and a dark shade in the same tray—so my clients can blend their own perfect shade. You can achieve the same results with other brands by selecting two shades of foundation that are no more than one-half to one shade different from each other. Use the five compacts shown here or the color smears on the opposite page as a guideline for combining shades.

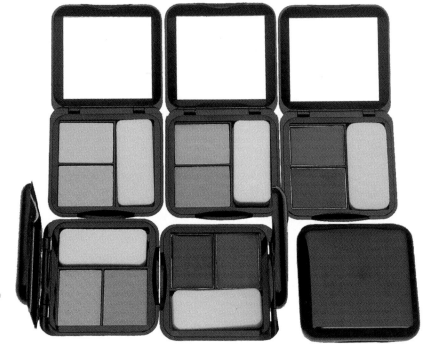

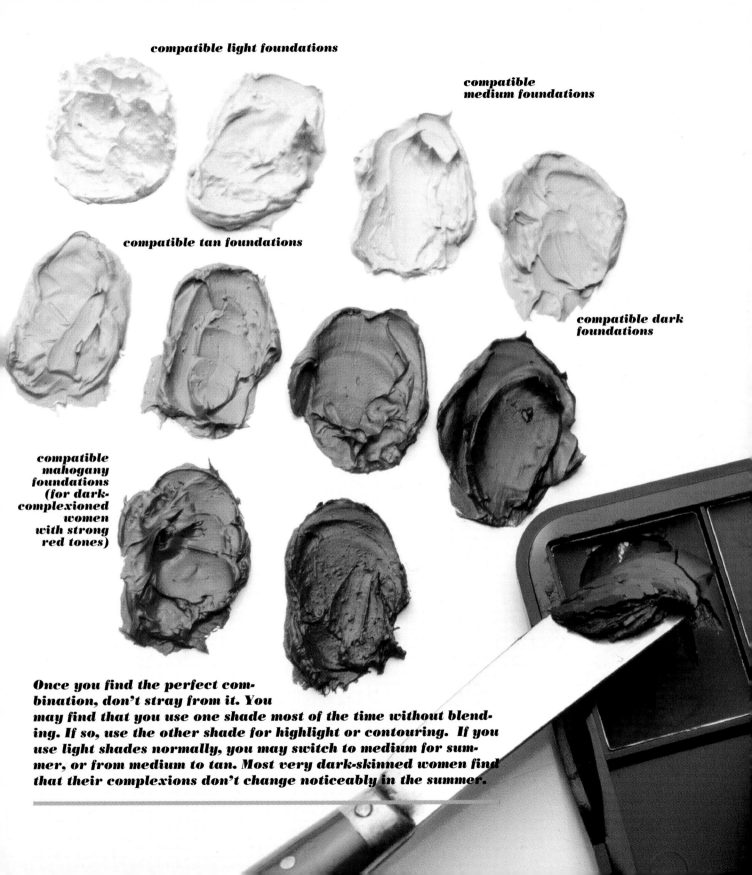

compatible light foundations

compatible medium foundations

compatible tan foundations

compatible dark foundations

compatible mahogany foundations (for dark-complexioned women with strong red tones)

Once you find the perfect combination, don't stray from it. You may find that you use one shade most of the time without blending. If so, use the other shade for highlight or contouring. If you use light shades normally, you may switch to medium for summer, or from medium to tan. Most very dark-skinned women find that their complexions don't change noticeably in the summer.

Foundation in Less Than a Minute

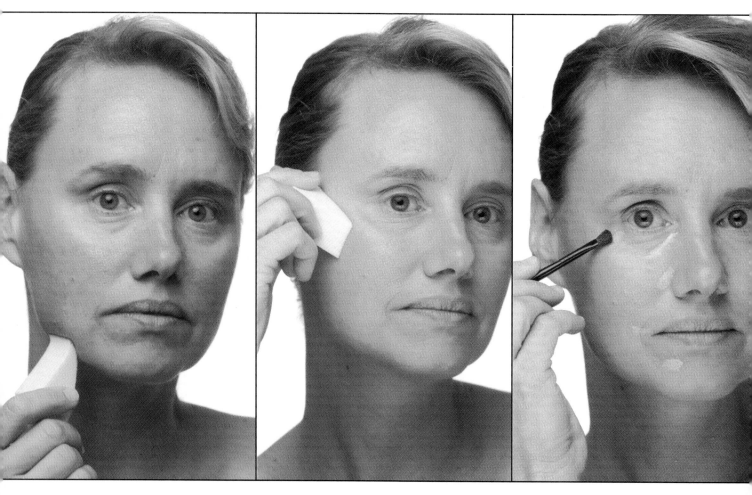

A sponge gives the most control when applying foundation. Dab the sponge into the foundation color (or colors) and apply to the jawline in a smooth, downward stroke, toward the chin.

After applying makeup on the jaw, under the jaw, and on the chin, use the sponge, in downward strokes, all over the face. Blend carefully under the lashes, around the nose and brows, and into the hairline

If there are dark areas under the eyes or around the nose, use a corrective brush to paint the shadows with a bit of foundation that is one-half to one shade lighter than what you've already applied. Blend lightly with the sponge.

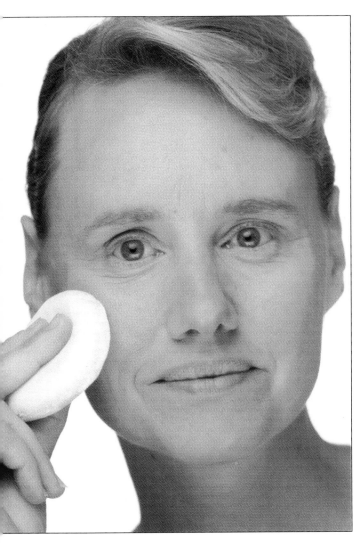

To finish, lightly powder your entire face with translucent powder. I use pressed powder applied with a puff rather than loose powder dusted on with a brush, but that's purely a personal preference (I feel that it's the easiest to control and the least messy).

Remember that a light veil of foundation is all that most women need to create a flawless finish. Once you've selected the right color and become adept at using a sponge, it should take less than a minute to apply your foundation. The four steps shown here will soon become second nature. I always recommend applying the foundation in downward strokes so the natural peach fuzz we all have stays smooth and unnoticeable.

Many women prefer not to wear foundation all over their faces. No problem—foundation can be used as a spot cover. Simply pick up a tiny bit of foundation with the sponge and dab color on a problem area (shadows, broken capillaries, scars or blemishes). Use a clean corner of the sponge to blend.

Sometimes it takes a heavier application to cover blemishes or scarring completely. Follow my four application steps. Before powdering, dab extra foundation on problem areas, blend again, and powder. Then go back with a powder puff (I occasionally spray the face lightly with my facial toner) and powder the problem areas again.

The Right Shade of Foundation for a No-Makeup Look

Remember—when it comes to foundation, less is always more. When foundation is visible, you lose the natural look.

There's nothing worse than seeing a woman who looks as if she's wearing a mask of beige gunk. That's too much foundation. If your skin is coated with foundation, use the sponge to remove the excess. Blend until your skin tone looks even but your natural texture is evident. If the sponge doesn't remove enough, use makeup remover and start over with a clean face. Just a bit of foundation, smoothed and blended with a sponge, creates a "less is more" natural sheen on your skin.

Other women make the mistake of trying to hide dark circles with light makeup. Wrong! That's when you end up with reverse-raccoon eyes—a white mask around your eyes that accentuates

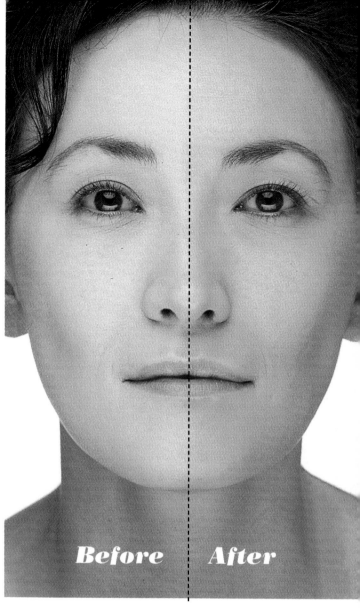

Before   After

Kaoru makes the mistake of using foundation that is too light and ends up looking as if she is wearing a mask. On the left in the photo above, her neck looks darker than her face. When she matches her base to her jawline, where face and neck meet, Kaoru achieves the perfect shade. Her skin tones are even, but she looks as if she's not wearing foundation.

problems rather than solving them. Using a foundation one-half to one shade lighter than the undereye circle will usually cover the darkened area and will blend easily with the rest of your foundation without leaving a line of demarcation.

Wearing a foundation that's too dark or too light will also create a masklike effect. As I noted earlier, the right foundation color makes all the difference. Refer to page 60 for tips on picking your best shade.

Improperly blended makeup is simple to take care of. Pull out your sponge and smooth it gently over your face in downward strokes. When you're finished, your skin should look evenly toned and there should be no line at the jaw where the foundation stops and your bare skin begins. You should never see sponge strokes. Properly applied foundation is perfectly sheer and smooth.

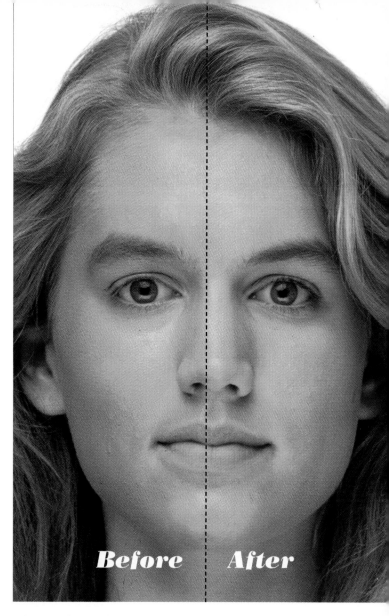

Before   After

Lisa, a beautiful teenager who mistakenly believed that everyone looks better tan, tried to achieve the sun-bronzed look with makeup that is too dark. Like Kaoru, she looks as if she's wearing a mask. The darker of her two medium foundations gives Lisa a healthy glow while still covering a few small blemishes. Just one shade darker than usual gives her a sun-kissed look.

How to Minimize Complexion Problems

Before

After

66

Trish has lines in her skin that makeup can minimize. Use a moisturizer to hydrate and plump the skin before applying foundation. After blending foundation, use a fine brush to paint lighter foundation in the creases. Dust lightly with powder. Gently go over the face with foundation sponge to eliminate extra powder.

When covering acne, opposite page, never try to camouflage blemishes with a light shade of heavy concealer. Instead, use foundation (if the spots are very pronounced, stipple over them with a shade one-half to one full shade lighter than your regular base), and blend the areas with foundation sponge. To finish, spritz the face with toner and press on powder with a puff.

Paula sometimes has puffiness under her eyes. Minimizing it requires foundation and great eye makeup. Apply full foundation. With a corrective brush apply a foundation one-half to one shade lighter in the deepest recess under the puff, then apply foundation one-half shade darker on top of the puff. Blend with sponge and powder to keep area matte. Strengthen area above eye with shadow and liner for balance.

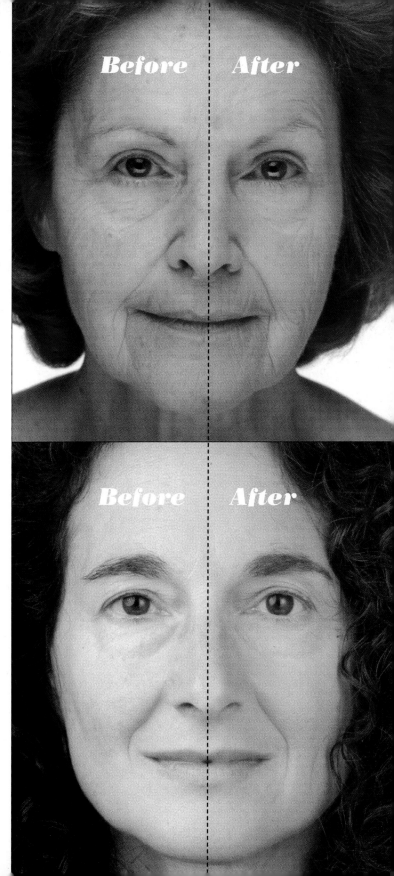

Before   After

Before   After

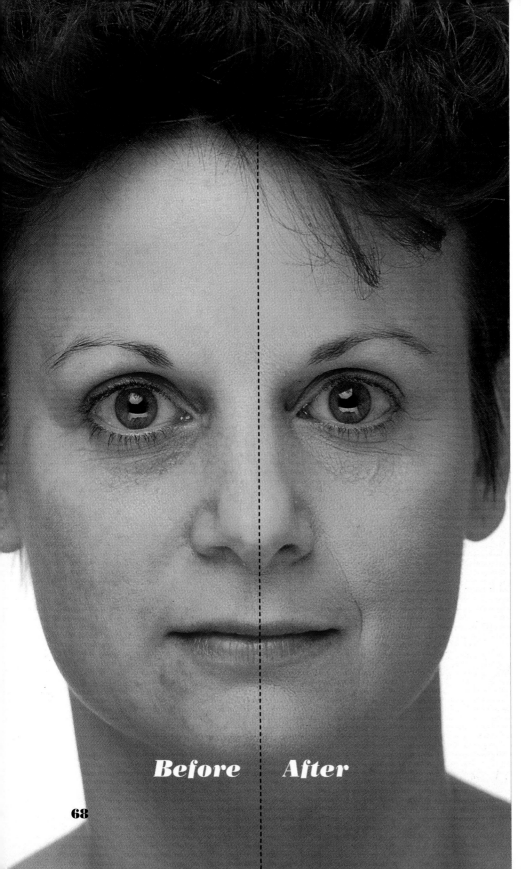

Before | **After**

Like so many women, Carol has dark circles under her eyes. To minimize, after applying base, use a corrective brush to apply a base that is about one-half to one shade lighter than the undereye circle. Use a very light touch with the brush, then follow with the sponge to blend.

Jaclyn has red spots on the side of her nose that bother her. That's a simple cover-up job for foundation. If one application doesn't cover a spot, after dusting with powder, go over the reddened areas with the foundation sponge and repowder. This technique works for scars and birthmarks.

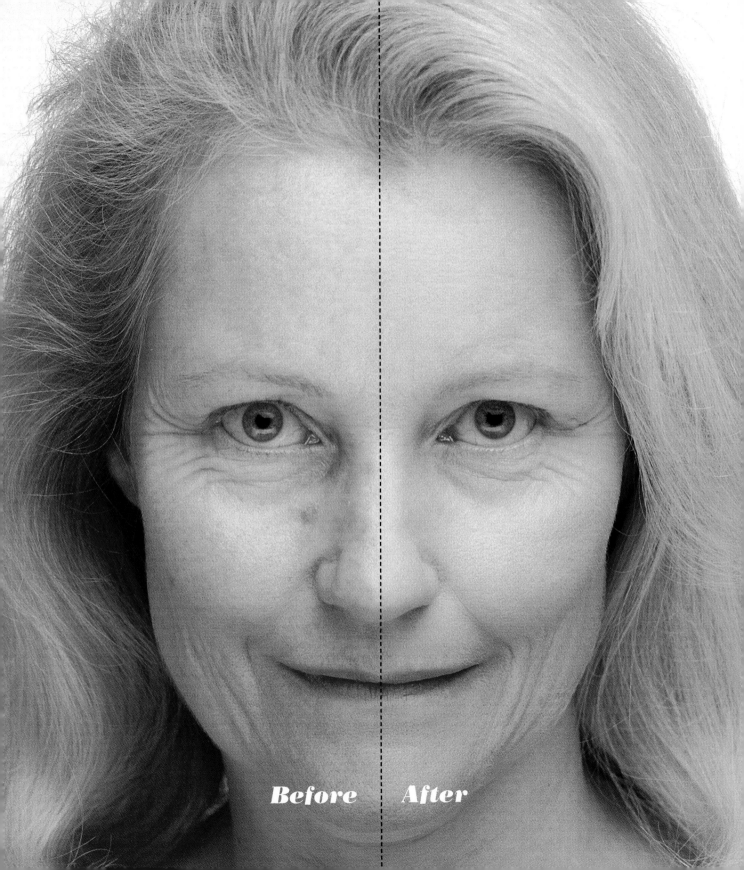

Before   *After*

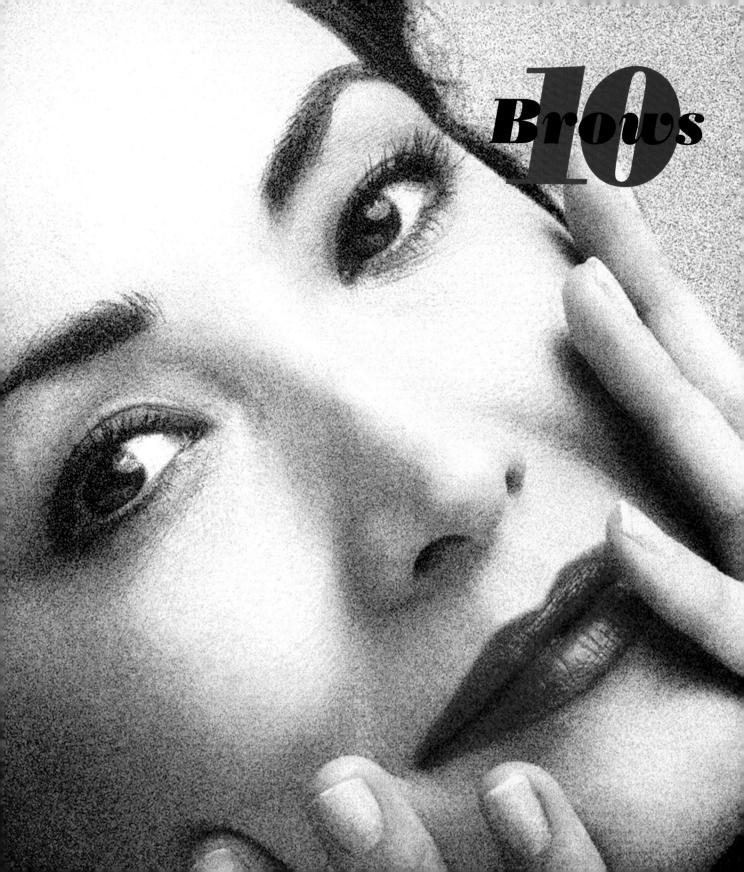

Eyebrows are the face's exclamation points. Everything the eyes communicate is emphasized by beautiful brows. Brows are also a means of subtly expressing your personal sense of style—they can be dramatic, tailored, or (the way I like them best) very natural.

What's more, the eyebrow is a way to keep up with fashion trends, since brow styles seem to shift frequently. Remember the 1950s brows that Marilyn Monroe and Elizabeth Taylor wore—full at the base and tapered to nothingness as they reached the temples? So shaped, so glamorous, so 1950s. In the 1960s brows started to fill out a bit, drifting away from the sophisticated, alluring look to a more innocent, natural brow à la Audrey Hepburn and Twiggy. Then, in the 1970s, women headed for the workplace, and the perfectly groomed brow fit right into the "dress for success" ethic. In the 1980s women assumed more power over their lives, and their brows became an emphatic statement of that power. Brooke Shields's beautiful furry eyebrows accented her all-around vitality as well as her

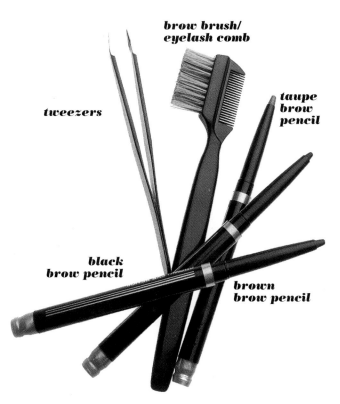

brow brush/
eyelash comb

tweezers

taupe
brow
pencil

black
brow pencil

brown
brow pencil

wonderful eyes. As we head into the twenty-first century, 1990s brows are gently contouring again with soft arches—refined and feminine symbols of fully emerged female confidence.

What these five decades of style indicate is that the average woman can look beautiful with almost any brow, as long as it is properly groomed. The best brows accentuate the eyes like a picture frame, complementing the color, the shape, and the expression. In the same way that an overpowering frame can detract from a canvas, a brow that calls attention to itself can minimize the impact of the eyes.

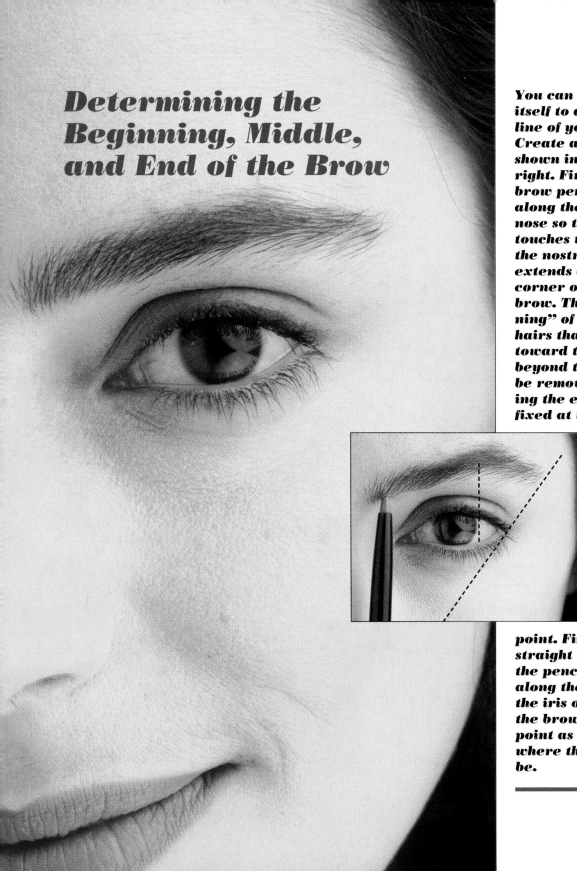

Determining the Beginning, Middle, and End of the Brow

You can use your eye itself to determine the line of your brow. Create a V shape as shown in the diagram at right. First hold your brow pencil vertically along the side of the nose so that one end touches the outside of the nostril and the point extends above the inner corner of your eye to the brow. That's the "beginning" of the brow; any hairs that are growing toward the middle beyond this point should be removed. Next, keeping the end of the pencil fixed at the bottom of the nostril, shift the point toward the outside corner of the eye and extend it to the brow. This is the "end" of the brow; pluck any hairs growing beyond this point. Finally, looking straight ahead, extend the pencil vertically along the outside edge of the iris of your eye to the brow; I think of this point as the "middle," or where the arch should be.

Grooming the Brow

Before you begin grooming your brows, select the correct tools. You can get by with three essentials—good tweezers, a brow brush or soft toothbrush, and a brow pencil. When I select tweezers, I prefer Tweezerman brand; they are expensive at about $20, but in my business their dependability is worth the investment. I've also been successful with Revlon tools, which are far more economical. I always choose the slant tip because it's easiest for me to work with, especially when I'm grasping fine hairs. It's certainly a personal preference. Just be sure the tweezers are in good condition so you can grasp the hair firmly and pull it out quickly by the root, without breaking it. As tweezers age the points fail to meet tightly no matter how hard you squeeze, so double-check. In fact, the harder you squeeze, the more the tweezers bend. With a good implement you shouldn't have to exert much pressure on the tool and the process should be quick and easy.

The brush is also matter of personal taste. I use a two-sided brush with a comb on one side, so it doubles as an eyelash separator. I choose natural bristles over the less expensive nylon styles—they're softer. As you will see, I use the brush several times during the makeup application process, so it's an important tool, well worth the initial investment. Many women are totally comfortable using a soft child-size toothbrush, although the bristles may be too wide for the finest line of a sculpted brow. Whatever brush you select, take care of it. I clean mine daily with a bit of eye makeup remover and a little soap, to remove any traces of oil, hairspray, and brow makeup. Then I store it like a toothbrush, so the bristles can air dry.

When it comes to a brow pencil, I'm devoted to my own brand, of course, but there are other fine pencils. Choose one with a very soft lead, so there's no drag on the skin. A rounded tip prevents harsh lines. The pencil should fit comfortably in your hand. I find that a long, slim pencil is easier to control than a fat, stubby one.

It often takes two shades of pencil to create a natural brow color. For most blondes and brunettes, I usually combine a few strokes each

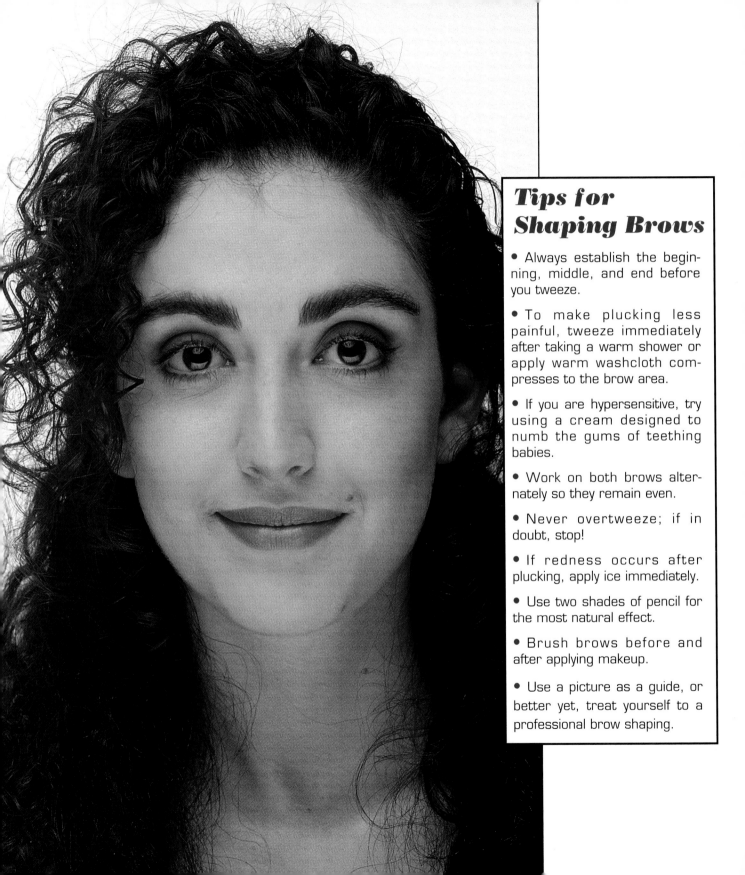

Tips for Shaping Brows

- Always establish the beginning, middle, and end before you tweeze.

- To make plucking less painful, tweeze immediately after taking a warm shower or apply warm washcloth compresses to the brow area.

- If you are hypersensitive, try using a cream designed to numb the gums of teething babies.

- Work on both brows alternately so they remain even.

- Never overtweeze; if in doubt, stop!

- If redness occurs after plucking, apply ice immediately.

- Use two shades of pencil for the most natural effect.

- Brush brows before and after applying makeup.

- Use a picture as a guide, or better yet, treat yourself to a professional brow shaping.

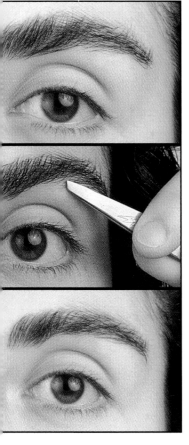

of taupe and brown. When the brows are naturally black, as with many ethnic women, I combine dark brown and taupe. Don't use black since it gives a very heavy and unnatural look to the brow. And for redheads, taupe is usually the best choice.

As a general guideline, select brow makeup that is a few shades lighter than your hair, unless you're a pale blonde, then go a shade or two darker. If your hair is gray, look for the color that is mixed with the gray (blond, brown, black, red), use the same guidelines listed above, but add a few gray strokes, too.

Tweezing Properly

If your brows need to be shaped, the best gift you can give yourself is a trip to a facial or beauty salon for a professional grooming. This service costs about $12 and is worth the price. After the brows have been shaped once, you can easily remove stray hairs as they begin growing in.

You *can* do it yourself. Just be sure to allow enough time to do a careful job. After you've removed hairs that stray from the natural beginning and end of your brows (as I explained on page 72), clean up the area between the brows. Then begin tweezing stray hairs under each brow. Rather than completing one brow and moving to the next, work a bit on each brow to make sure the brows stay even. Many people will tell you not to remove hairs from the tops of your brows. I disagree. But proceed with caution—just tweeze the hairs that grow above the natural line of the brows, not those that create fullness.

Natural Brows

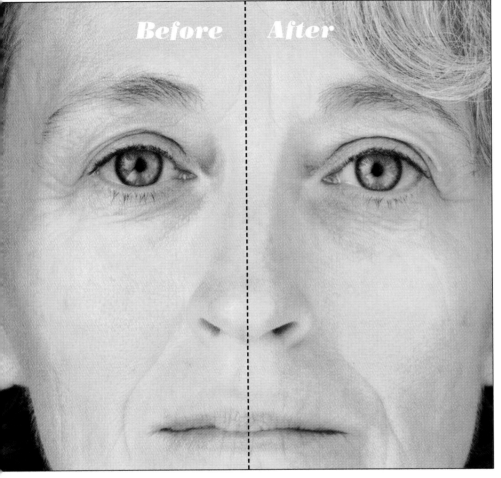

Before | After

Just a few strokes of taupe brow pencil is all that Gloria needs for a very natural-looking brow. She follows the natural line; she fills in a bit at the beginning, middle, and end, then brushes the brows well to accent their fullness.

Gloria has nicely shaped brows that add character to her face. I'm using her to illustrate an important point: Some women look in the mirror, see brows like Gloria's, and try to change them. These are great brows! Don't fool with them. Notice that the brows begin just above the inner corner of her eye and extend slightly beyond the outer corner— exactly the right proportion for her face. All she needed to do was remove stray hairs without trying to alter the shape. They're dark enough that she doesn't need much brow makeup. A bit of brushing and perhaps a bit of clear mascara keeps them shiny. When she does want to wear makeup, a bit of taupe pencil will strengthen her brows while keeping the overall effect very natural.

Overplucked Brows

Many times teenagers get carried away with their tweezers and end up with skimpy brows when they get older. Overplucked brows like Carol's don't look natural and don't adequately accent her beautiful eyes. Nearest the nose, where brows are usually thicker, hers are thin. Instead of beginning above the inner corner of her eye, Carol's brow begins above the inner edge of her iris. The effect is that her eyes look too close together, when actually they are well spaced. A minor correction with brow makeup changes the illusion. By darkening her brow a bit and adding more fullness near the bridge of the nose, they seem less sparse, but she doesn't end up with a painted-on look.

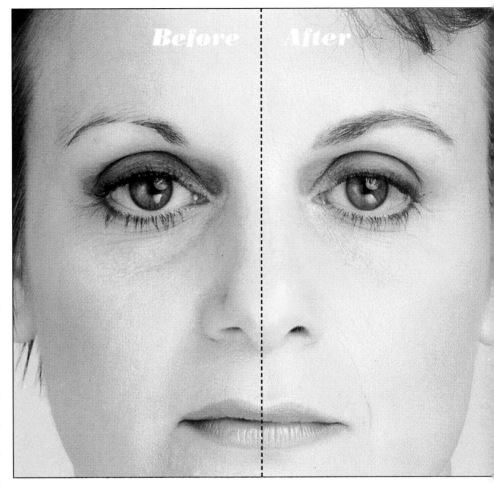

Before *After*

The most important step to enhance Carol's overplucked brows is to thicken the beginning of the brow. To make it look fuller near the bridge of the nose, Carol applies short strokes of color, both taupe and brown above and below the existing brow and a few wispy strokes toward the nose. After adding some fullness, she can follow the natural line of the brow to the end.

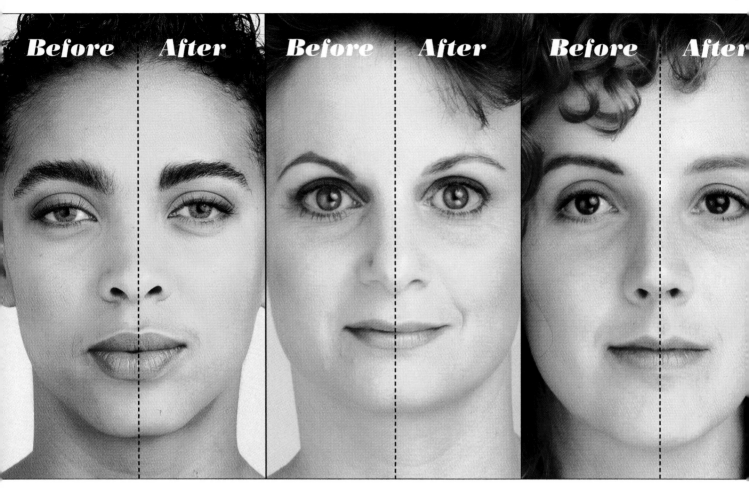

Before **After**   **Before** **After**   **Before** **After**

Brows Too Full

Wendy's brows are beautiful, just a bit too full and overpowering. Removing a few hairs underneath the brow creates a more controlled and refined look.

Arch Too Sharp

Carol tried to add strength to her brows by emphasizing the arch but she ended up with a harsh, unnatural look. Darkening her natural brow and adjusting the width is all she really needs.

Makeup Too Heavy

Sydney has such beautiful red hair. That heavy dark brown brow pencil looks totally unnatural with her hair. By using a lighter taupe pencil, she doesn't let her brow call attention to itself.

78

Applying Eyebrow Makeup

Once you've shaped your brows, makeup adds definition. If your brows are sparse in places, too thin all over, too short, or too shapeless, you can enhance them with a brow pencil. Always keep in mind that the goal is a natural-looking brow, not something that looks drawn on.

The reason I use a very soft pencil is that it easily deposits color on the skin and brow hairs. Use short, wispy strokes. Apply the strokes between the natural hairs, drawing them in the same direction the hairs grow. Never outline the brow and try to fill it in—nothing looks more artificial! Trying to simulate a hair with a hard, pointy pencil usually results in a very hard, unnatural look. Once you've applied the pencil, use a brow brush to blend the strokes. Brush the brows up, smooth the top edge in the direction brows grow.

I always suggest that your brows be colored before applying eye makeup so the proportion is appropriate to your face. It may look as though your brow makeup is too heavy, but that will change when you add eye makeup. After you've finished the eye makeup, recheck your brows. If they need to be toned down, simply brush a little more with your brow brush. If they need to be strengthened, add a bit more pencil. Now's the time to add a fine coat of clear mascara to keep brows in place. If you prefer, a bit of soap or hairspray on the brow brush will also tame wild brows. For a dramatic evening look, try applying a coat of dark brown or black mascara. Remember: brows should never overpower your eyes.

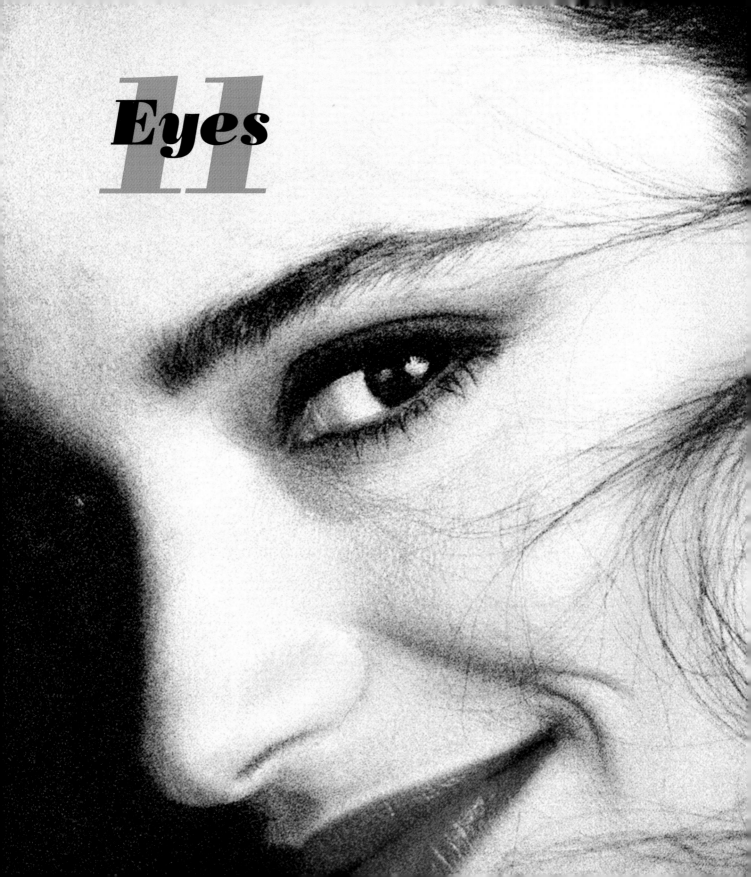

Eyes

11

*L*ook in the mirror—no eye makeup, please. Now study your eyes. Aren't they fantastic? I can guarantee you that they are beautiful; everybody's eyes are wonderful when you look into them. Eyes are the quintessential beauty signature, no matter what color or shape they are.

There's no such thing as the "perfect" eye. Don't get stuck in old patterns, thinking that eyes have to be huge, almond-shaped, and perfectly spaced to be pretty. On the next several pages you'll see all kinds of eyes. And believe me, they're all remarkable.

In the same way that I believe every eye is beautiful, I firmly believe that every eye looks better with some makeup. Yes, many women look wonderful with no eye makeup, but they look better with a subtle addition of mascara, liner, or shadow. Or all three.

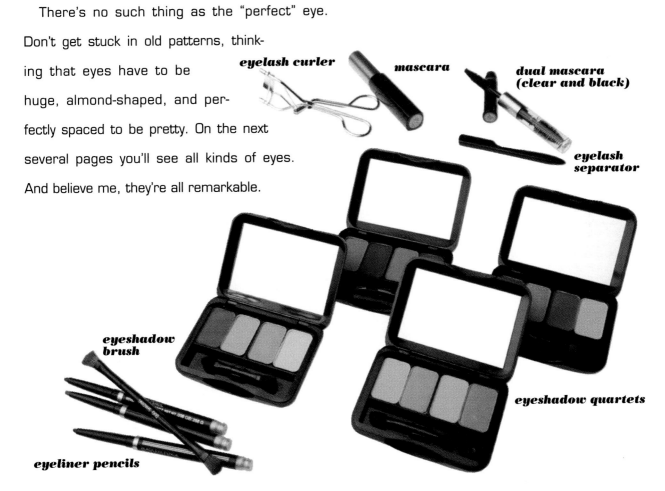

eyelash curler

mascara

dual mascara (clear and black)

eyelash separator

eyeshadow brush

eyeshadow quartets

eyeliner pencils

I would never suggest that anyone try to dramatically change the look of their eyes with cosmetics. It doesn't work. I hate walking into a department store and seeing the models' faces loaded with a rainbow of "the newest spring shades" of eye makeup. You don't see their eyes; you see their makeup. Most of the time you probably wouldn't be able to recall the color of the model's eyes—instead you would remember the color of her company's newest eye shadow. The makeup becomes the statement, not the woman's unique beauty. That's not my style, and I hope it's not yours. Eyes should communicate for you, not advertise your makeup.

However, shadows, liner, and mascara in subtle colors can achieve two important goals. First, they enhance the eyes, making the natural color appear more intense and the lashes longer and lusher. Second, the makeup helps the eyes look bigger, something most of us find desirable.

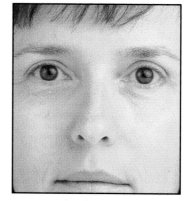

Small Eyes

Before

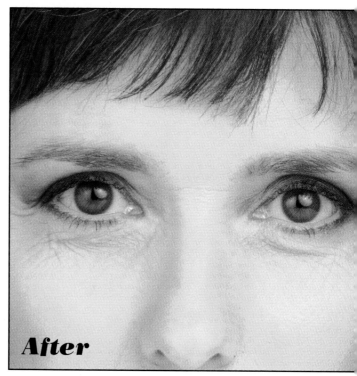

After

Kathleen's eyes are small in proportion to the size of her face, but they're quite attractive. Since she has other delicate features—a slim nose and fine lips—her eyes are consistent with her refined look. Makeup makes her eyes look larger and more dramatic. However, too much shadow and liner will make them look smaller. Here's where good placement and blending are extremely important.

Intensifying the color and making the eyes look bigger doesn't alter the inherent shape or position of the eyes. I think it's much more interesting to play up the unique look of your eyes. That's not to say that Luanne, photographed on page 86, would want to concentrate all of her shadow near her nose in an attempt to make her close-set eyes appear closer together. But, neither would she try to make her eyes look farther apart. By making her eyes look their best—bigger and brighter—she will call attention to their beauty, and that's all that matters. No one will notice that her eyes are close-set. Darwyn, photographed at right, has quite prominent eyes. I've heard make-up artists use negative terms like "bulging" and talk about ways to "set them back" or "make them recede." No way. She can make her beautiful eyes even more dramatic and balance them with gorgeous lips.

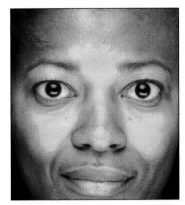

Prominent Eyes

Before

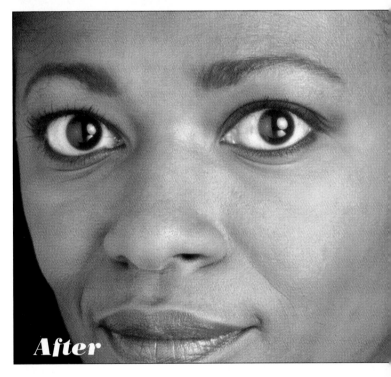

After

Darwyn's eyes are large and dominate her face. Because of their sheer size, large eyes can look overly made up without careful makeup placement. Part of enhancing them is establishing a balance on the face. If the eye makeup is strong, the lips should be equally strong. If the eye makeup is pale, or the eye is bare, a muted lipstick will create balance. Here Darwyn uses brown liner under the lashes of her lower lid and dark brown shadow on the lid, without extending it up and out toward the temple.

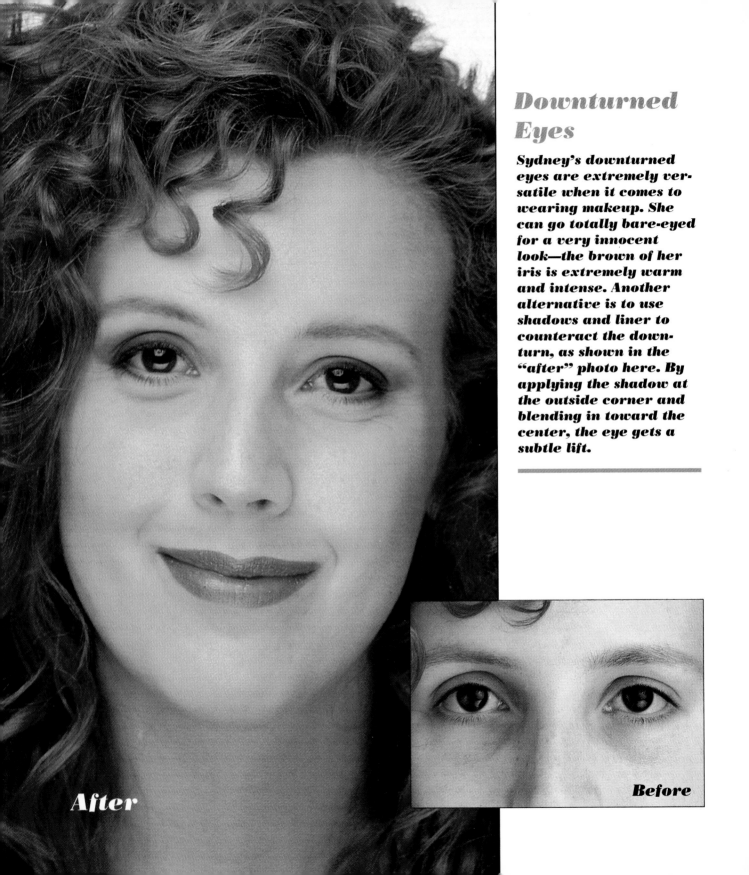

Downturned Eyes

Sydney's downturned eyes are extremely versatile when it comes to wearing makeup. She can go totally bare-eyed for a very innocent look—the brown of her iris is extremely warm and intense. Another alternative is to use shadows and liner to counteract the downturn, as shown in the "after" photo here. By applying the shadow at the outside corner and blending in toward the center, the eye gets a subtle lift.

After

Before

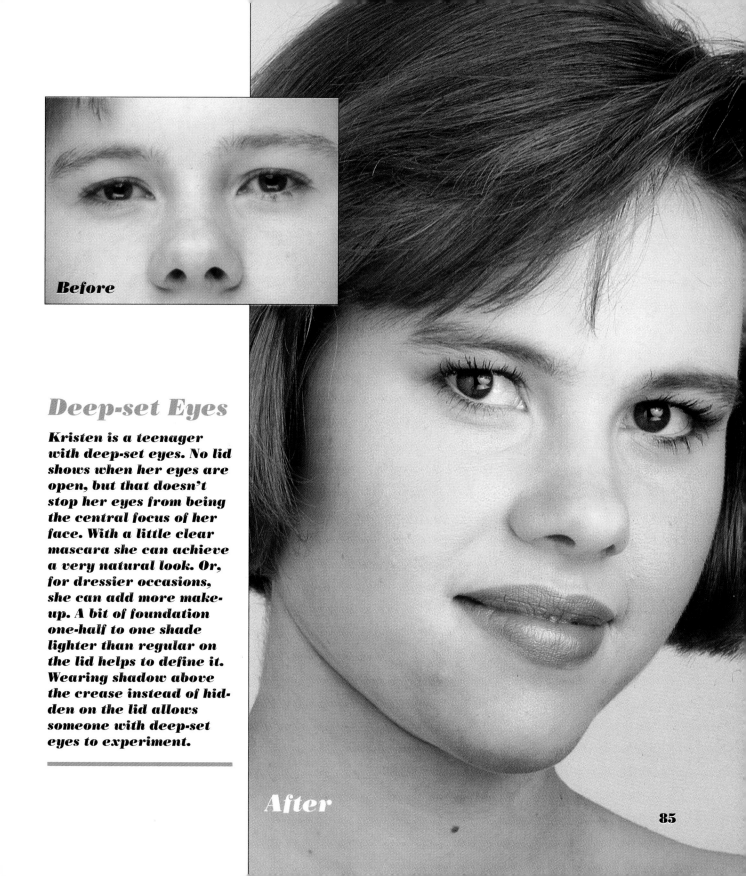

Before

Deep-set Eyes

Kristen is a teenager with deep-set eyes. No lid shows when her eyes are open, but that doesn't stop her eyes from being the central focus of her face. With a little clear mascara she can achieve a very natural look. Or, for dressier occasions, she can add more make-up. A bit of foundation one-half to one shade lighter than regular on the lid helps to define it. Wearing shadow above the crease instead of hidden on the lid allows someone with deep-set eyes to experiment.

After

85

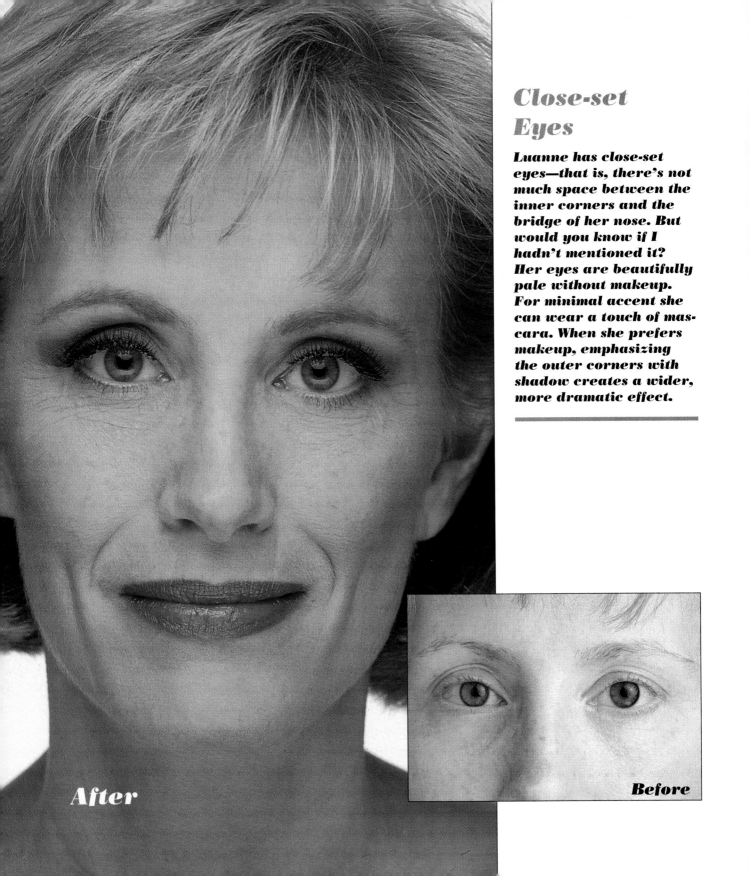

Close-set Eyes

Luanne has close-set eyes—that is, there's not much space between the inner corners and the bridge of her nose. But would you know if I hadn't mentioned it? Her eyes are beautifully pale without makeup. For minimal accent she can wear a touch of mascara. When she prefers makeup, emphasizing the outer corners with shadow creates a wider, more dramatic effect.

After

Before

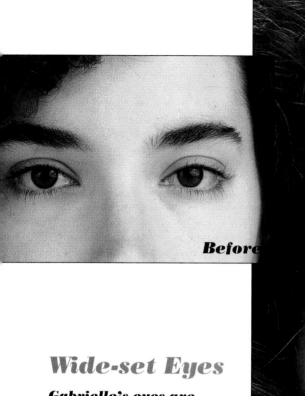

Before

Wide-set Eyes

Gabrielle's eyes are wide-set—there's more than the usual space between the inside corners and the bridge of the nose. She has a wonderful doe-eyed look that works well with or without makeup. Because she has dark lashes, she doesn't need mascara unless she uses it after curling her lashes to set them. When she wears more makeup, playing up the inner corners treats her wide-set eyes as an asset.

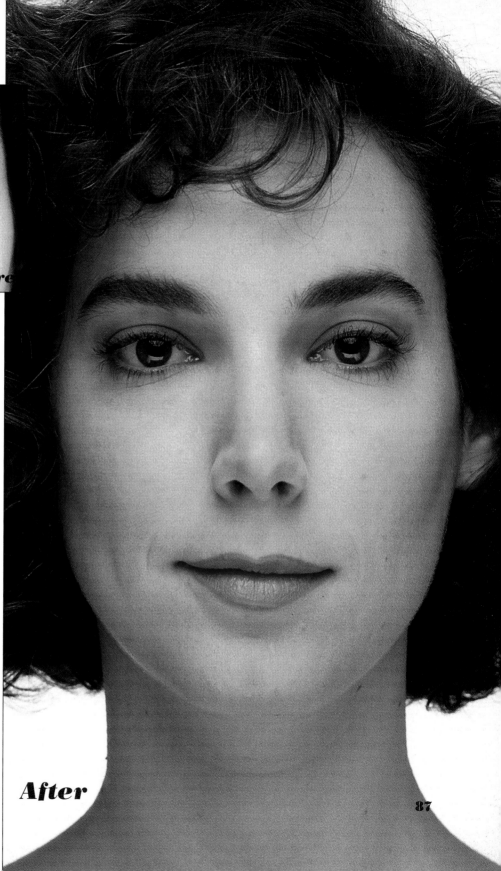

After

87

Applying Eye Shadow

Applying shadows takes three quick steps. Remember: Use a maximum of three colors at once: light, medium, and dark shades that blend well.

● **Step 1: Establish the outer corner first. Apply medium shade in a ">" shape and blend toward center of lid.**

● **Step 2: Add lighter shade to inner corner and blend with the medium shade.**

Tip: Applying foundation to the lid first will keep your eye makeup fresher longer.

● **Step 3: Apply darker shade at lash line on outside corner and blend into ">" and into crease. Blend.**

Tip: Start applying shadow at outer corner and work in—not vice versa. This method deposits the most color near the outer corner and makes the eye look bigger.

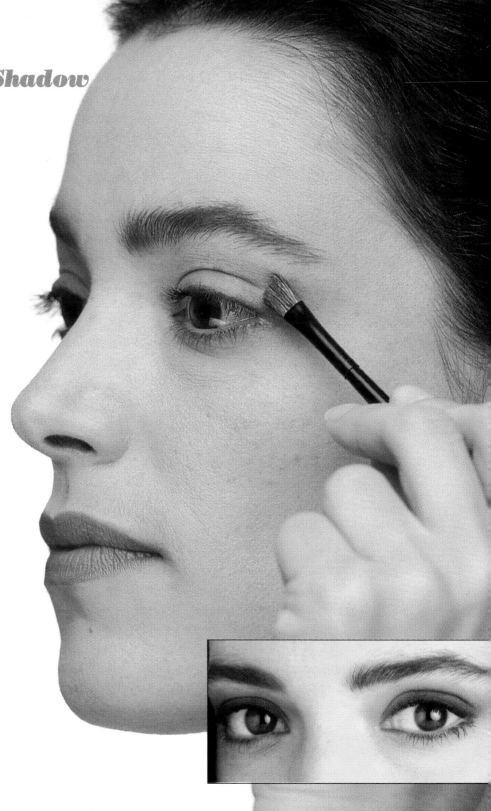

Choosing Shadow Colors

Selecting shadows is a way to express your moods and creativity. I hope you're not feeling locked in to a particular color palette because you've been told you that you are a certain "season." I like to encourage experimentation, as long as the color of the shadow enhances the color of your iris.

Don't match your shadow to your eye color (or your outfit—that looks old-fashioned). Instead, match unusual flecks of color in the irises. Brown and gray are universally popular shadows—most eyes have tiny dots of brown and gray. Many brown eyes also have traces of warm gold, red, green, and violet. That's why brown eyes look great with almost any shadow. Blue eyes often have cool green, lavender, and turquoise specks, so those shades bring out the iris. Medium or pale blue shadows detract from it. Green and hazel irises often show traces of palest gray and turquoise or gold and dark brown. Shadows of light or medium greens detract.

For the most versatility, select a complementary palette of light, medium, and dark shades, and you can add a fourth color as an accent. Some compatible combinations are shown at right.

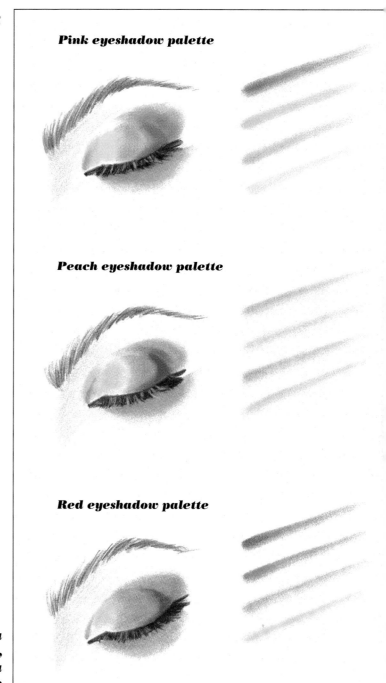

Pink eyeshadow palette

Peach eyeshadow palette

Red eyeshadow palette

Eyeliner and Mascara

I provide separate instructions for applying shadow because some women only wear liner and mascara. If you use everything, the liner goes on after the shadow. Mascara is the final step.

On the upper lid, use a soft eye pencil to draw a line from the inner corner to the outer corner, as close to lashes as possible. The line should be thicker toward the outer corner.

On the lower lid, under the lashes, start at the outside corner and draw a line that extends about two-thirds of the way toward the inner corner. Smudge the line with your fingertip or sponge.

Curl upper lashes with an eyelash curler, squeezing it closed for 10 to 20 seconds (this step is optional). Apply a coat of clear or black mascara; let it dry. That's enough for a no-makeup look. For lusher lashes, follow with another coat of black mascara. Comb lashes. Let dry. Repeat. Hold mascara wand vertically, coat lower lashes; comb. Remove residue under lashes with Q-Tip.™

All women can follow the eye make-up application steps on pages 88 and 90, but different types of eyes require slight variations in shadow and liner placement, so I've included those modifications here. In all cases, apply mascara as directed on page 90.

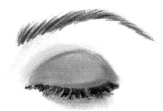

Prominent Eyes

Select matte shadows, never iridescent. Use medium shade to form "<" in outer corners, but do not extend eye. Blend medium or dark shade on lid and under brow bone. Line upper lid; smudge. Line lower lid from outer corner to center, keeping line as close to the roots of lower lashes as possible; smudge.

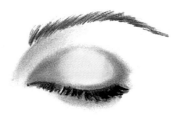

Wide-set Eyes

Establish "<" in outer corner with medium shade as directed on page 88. Blend medium shade on lid up to brow bone and toward center of lid. Blend darkest shade on lid at inner corner, first up toward brow, then toward middle of lid. Add lightest shade in center of lid and blend. Line upper lid. Line lower lid with taupe on outer half, brown or black on inner half.

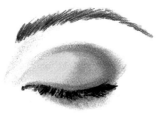

Hooded Eyes

Follow step 1 on page 88, using darkest shadow. Blend over hood, extending "<" to brow bone. (Don't close eye—look straight in the mirror, hold skin above eye taut, and apply shadow.) Blend medium shade on center of lid, up toward brow. Apply lightest shade on inner corner of lid. Line top lid and one-third of outer lower lid. Smudge lines.

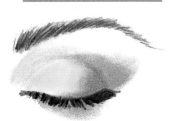

Downturned Eyes

When following step 1 on page 88, adjust "<" so its point angles up. Blend dark shade on outer third of lid only. Blend lightest shade on inner corner of lid, up into brow. Add medium shade only in center of lid at crease and blend up to brow bone. Blend well. When lining upper lid, stop short of outer corner. Line outer three-fourths of lower lid. Smudge lines, especially at outer corners.

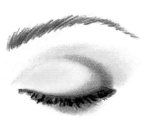

Small Eyes

Used medium shade to form "<" in outer corners. Blend shadow over entire lid and past "<" to extend eye. Accent "<" with darkest shade and blend into crease and into medium shade. Add lightest shade in corners. Line upper lid and outer third of lower lid. Smudge both lines.

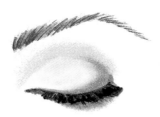

Deep-set Eyes

Follow directions on page 88. At step 2, use medium shadow or lighter shadow on lids. Blend lightest shade in middle of lid and up toward brow. Line upper lid. Line outer third of lower lashes and smudge both lines.

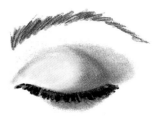

Close-set Eyes

Use lightest shadow on inner half of lid; darker shade on outer corner; blend outward. Follow basic directions on page 88. Then blend darkest shade from middle of lid up to brow bone and out toward outer corners. When applying liner, only line outer two-thirds of upper lid and outer half of lower lids.

Eye Makeup Mistakes

Too Much Liner

Luanne is wearing too much dark eyeliner on the left side of this photo. The first things anyone noticed when they looked at her were those huge rings of black around a relatively pale green eye. Part of what's beautiful about her eyes is the delicate color. That dark makeup worked in the late 1960s and 1970s, when the style for young women was heavy eye makeup. Now the dark line not only looks dated, it makes her face appear hard and tired. With a smudged soft brown liner, the true color of her iris predominates. Her eye makeup looks more contemporary and natural.

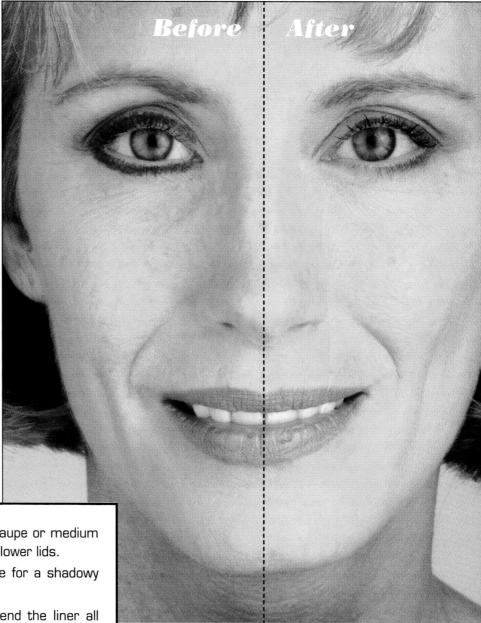

Before   After

Tips

- Instead of black liner, use taupe or medium brown on both the upper and lower lids.
- Be sure to smudge the line for a shadowy effect.
- On the lower lid, don't extend the liner all the way to the inner corner.

Too Much Makeup and the Wrong Shade

Here are two common makeup mistakes working against Gloria's eyes. Either one would be a problem individually, but together the're a disaster. On the "before" side, Gloria has too much makeup on her eye and it's the wrong color. Using a blue eyeshadow is the wrong choice for her—it detracts from the beautiful blue of her eyes. And instead of downplaying wrinkles and crinkles, the excess makeup exaggerates them. Applying a muted neutral shade accentuates the blue iris. Notice how much brighter her eye looks when she wears less shadow in this flattering shade.

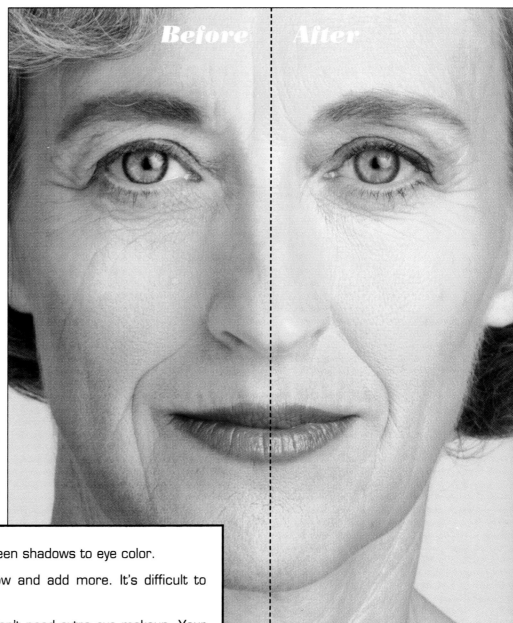

Before | After

Tips

- Avoid matching blue or green shadows to eye color.

- Start with minimal shadow and add more. It's difficult to take color off once it's on.

- If you wear glasses, you don't need extra eye makeup. Your frames will accent, and sometimes magnify, your eyes.

Poor Placement

Eye makeup worn in the wrong spots can ruin the look of a beautiful eye. In the "before" photo, Sydney tried to alter the shape of her downturned eyes with shadow. The result was that they looked overly made up and unnatural. She can achieve her goal with much less makeup—the shadows are concentrated in the corners and angled up slightly. The upward strokes of shadow seem to "lift" the outer corners of her eye.

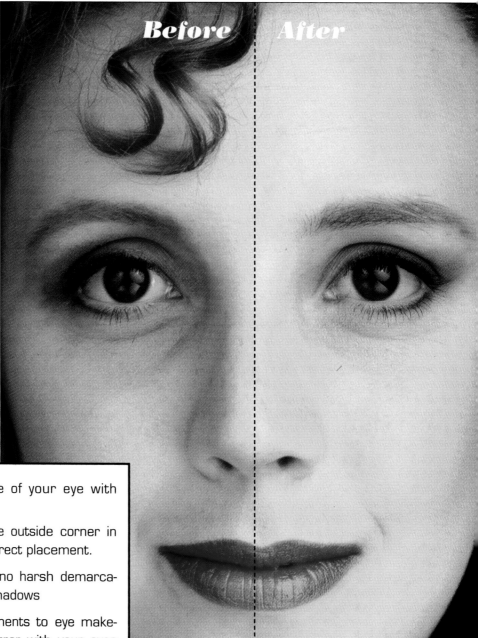

Before **After**

Tips

• Accent the natural shape of your eye with liner.

• Applying shadows from the outside corner in immediately helps set the correct placement.

• Blend carefully so there's no harsh demarcation between dark and light shadows

• When making final adjustments to eye make-up, look straight into the mirror with your eyes open naturally. Strengthen or minimize shadows with your eye in this position.

Iridescent Shadow

There's a place for iridescent shadow, but not on Trish. Iridescent shadow looks terrific on young girls determined to have some fun with their makeup and on fashion models making a visual statement in a photograph. But for the average woman over 30, iridescent shadow accents everything that might be wrong with the eye. The only time I suggest a sparkly shadow is for a very special evening occasion. And even then, use just a touch as an accent— never cover the whole lid. In the "after" photo, Trish's eye makeup follows my basic steps and looks much more natural.

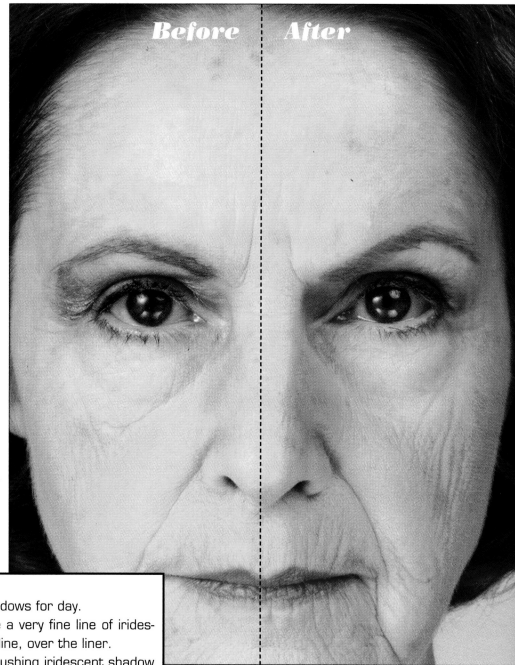

Before   After

Tips

- Never wear iridescent shadows for day.
- For special occasions use a very fine line of iridescent shadow along the lash line, over the liner.
- For a special effect, try brushing iridescent shadow on your lashes over a coat of clear mascara.

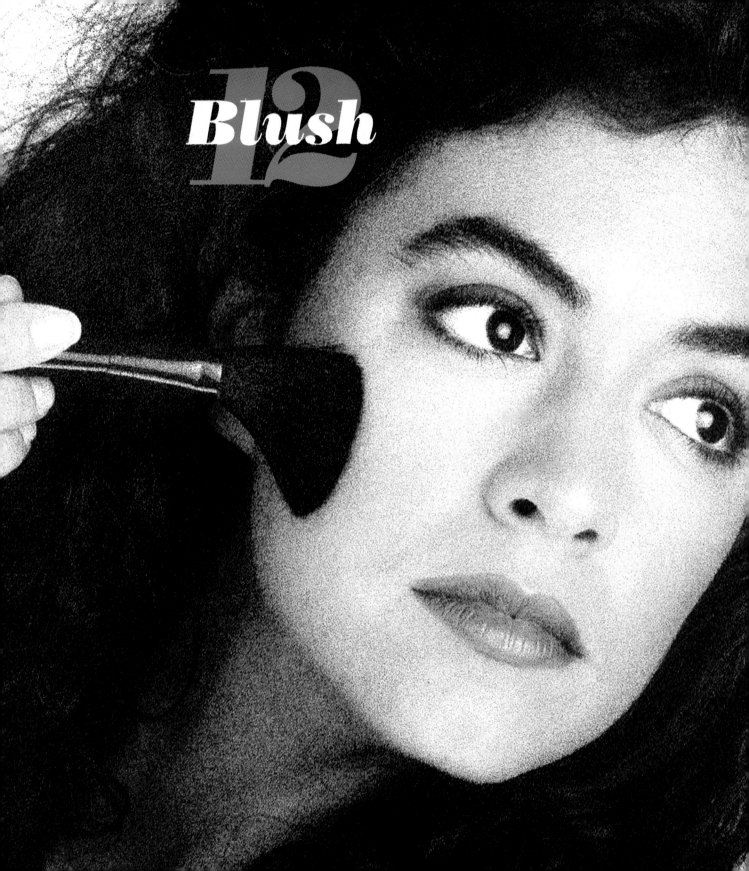

12 Blush

Blush is the "feel good" part of the makeup process. Blush adds a glow to your face, even when you're not feeling any sparkle. It provides a touch of cheek color that makes every woman look healthier and more vibrant.

I definitely depend on blush to make a difference in the way I appear. Like you, there are days when I'm overstressed, and my face is the first place that shows it. I'm drained, I look washed out, and I need a little lift. That's when I pull out my blush.

Rouging the cheeks has been a beauty secret through the ages. Frescoes showed the early Egyptians with reddish stains on their cheeks, and legend has it that Cleopatra used berry juices to affect a natural blush. During this century, trends in cheek makeup have shifted as often as hemlines. Flappers wore clownish circles of rouge in the 1920s, a look that continued into the 1930s. Then, in the 1940s and 1950s, those apple cheeks faded to a softer, more natural look. The revolution came in the 1960s and 1970s when powdered blush replaced cream rouge as the cheek makeup of choice. Wielding a wide brush and dark powder, women opted to carve artificial hollows in their cheeks with harsh stripes of blush. Now the look is subtle and natural—a refreshing change.

Remember that blush defines the inherent structure of your face. It accentuates everything that's beautiful about you. On the next several pages you'll see what a difference blush makes.

Compatible Blush Pairs

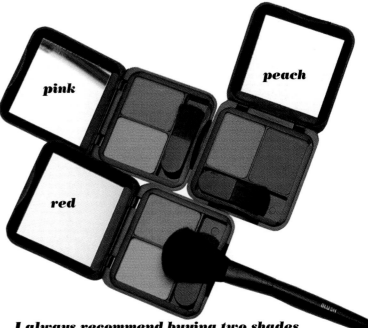

I always recommend buying two shades of blush: one for defining, and contouring, one for highlighting. Here are compatible combinations for use with peach, pink, and red lipsticks.

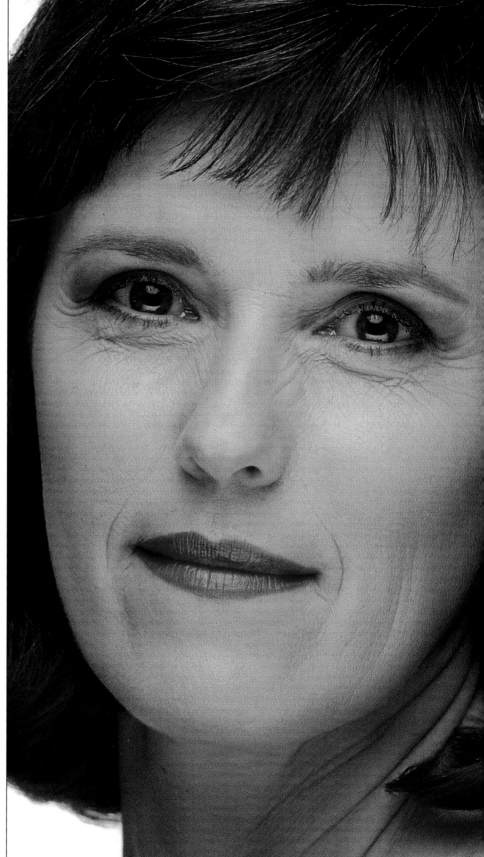

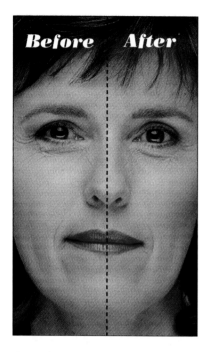

Before **After**

Kathleen looks fine without any makeup at all, but a bit of color helps adds contour to her face. Like so many women, Kathleen doesn't have cheekbones that are strong and angular. On the right side above, notice how blush adds definition and helps to emphasize her eyes.

Applying Blush

The most common question I hear about make-up is, "Where does the blush go?" I don't blame you if you're confused. I was, too, until I realized that all the chatter about various face shapes is irrelevant. Find the best blush placement this way: Use your fingers to locate the joint where upper and lower jaws meet. Your cheekbone starts there. Trace the bone downward until you feel a natural hollow. Apply darkest blush under this bone, starting in the hollow. To find the "apple," smile at the mirror; the fullest part of the cheek is the "apple." Light blush goes here.

Tips for Applying Blush

- Always complete eye makeup before applying blush. When your eyes are done, you won't feel the need for as much blush.

- Use two shades of blush—the lightest goes on the apple of the cheek, the darker under the cheekbone

- Apply the blush very lightly at first—add more when your makeup is complete, if necessary.

- If you've applied too much, use your foundation sponge to blend away the excess.

- Always blend thoroughly—nothing looks worse than an obvious stripe of blush.

- Blush should always fade completely into the hairline.

Here's my C key to applying blush. Use dark shade first. Start application in natural hollow. With one smooth stroke, make a "C" shape up toward the temple and hairline. Then, smile and apply light shade on the "apple" of your cheek.

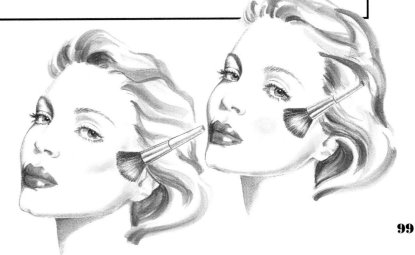

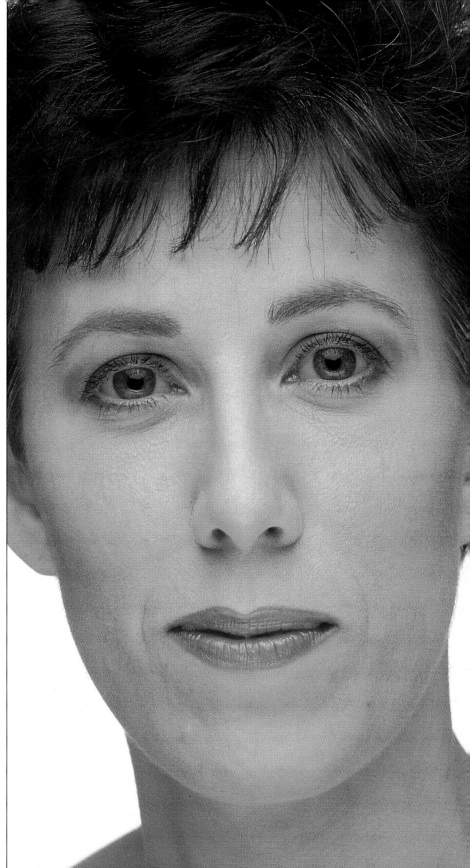

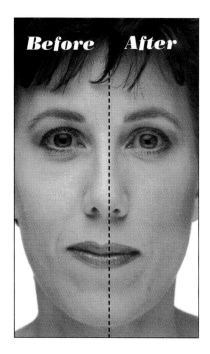

Laura has a long face, and since she likes to deemphasize its length, her fluffy short haircut with its wispy bangs does wonders to help change the geometry. Notice how, on the right side of the photo above, the addition of blush immediately calls attention to her eyes.

Long Face

You can take two approaches with a long face—emphasize its length or use blush to add width. The first is very dramatic, with very little makeup—maybe just a touch of eyeliner and mascara, a bold shiny lipstick, no blush—hair slicked back. Most women, however, like a softer look.

To achieve it, add a light shade of blush on top of your cheekbones and a darker shade under the bone. Focus most of the color on the outer edges of the bone, where the jaws meet, and up, toward the temple. Bangs or soft waves on the forehead help shorten the look of the face, too.

Tips for a Long Face

- Using two shades of blush will highlight the cheekbones and widen the face.
- Apply blush low on the temple, never higher than the tip of the eyebrows.
- When adding light blush on top of cheekbones, don't get too close to the under-eye area or they'll look puffy.
- Keep forehead and chin free of blush so attention is focused on eyes and lips.
- A dusting of light blush on the tip of the nose will highlight the center of the face.

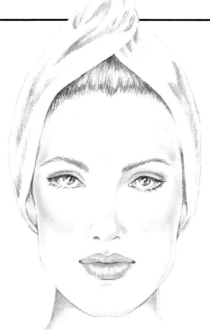

See page 99 for blush placement. Apply darkest blush in a "C," as noted. Concentrate color at the outer edge of face—the middle of the "C" and up toward the temple. Add lighter shade above cheekbone and blend. Dust the light shade on the "apple."

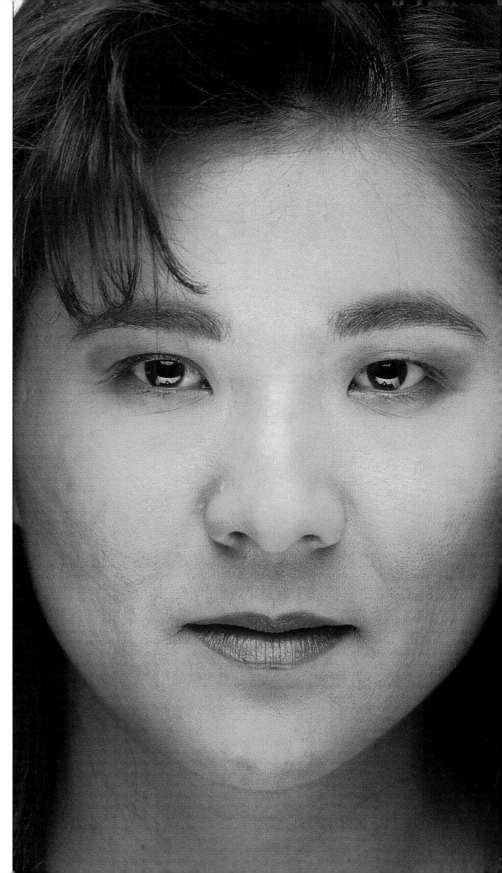

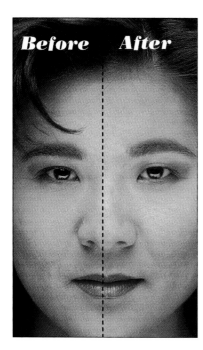

Before   After

Lisa's wide face some-
times gives her the illu-
sion of being chubby,
despite the fact that
she's slim. She uses blush
to narrow her face. In
the photo above, the
blush on the right side of
the photo, accentuates
her cheeks and adds
streamlined angles.

102

Wide Face

Whether you've been born with a wide face or are a few pounds heavier than usual, blush can slim your face. Or, if you prefer, you can apply blush in a way that does not exaggerate the width of the face but doesn't downplay it, either. Both approaches can be very attractive. Be confident knowing that full cheeks look more youthful in real life than the photogenic sunken cheeks of high-fashion models (and skeletons). Making the most of your cheeks depends on the interplay of carefully blended light and dark blushes to create the illusion of natural angles.

Tips for a Wide Face

- Keep the blush shades concentrated high on the cheekbone and on the "apple."

- Never apply the blush higher than your eyes on the temple.

- Don't apply blush too close to your nose or your features will seem crowded together.

- Rather than using dark contouring powders, which tend to look artificial, try dusting your blush brush with brown eye shadow before dipping into the blush. The two powders will blend to a create a slightly darker blush.

- Blend carefully or you'll see stripes of light and dark color on your face—the illusion will be gone.

- Add a bit of the light blush to the tip of your chin.

See page 99 for blush placement. Apply darkest blush in a "C," as noted. Concentrate color in the hollow of the cheeks and do not use blush high on the temples. To slim the face, apply a lighter color on top of the cheekbone, under the dark blush and on the "apple." Blend carefully.

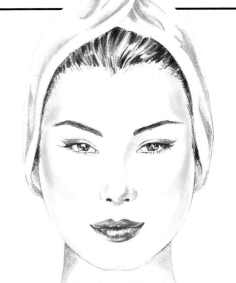

Common Blush Mistakes

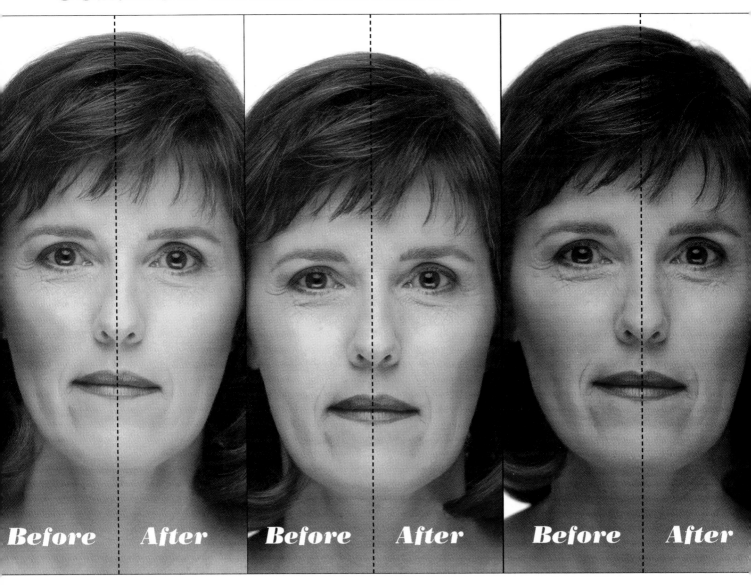

Before   After   Before   After   Before   After

The left side of the photo above shows Kathleen wearing too much blush. She looks as if she is totally unskilled at makeup application. On the right, she's wearing just enough.

On the left side of the photo above, Kathleen's blush placement is off. Too high, it intrudes on the eye region and makes her eye look puffy. On the right the blush is perfectly positioned.

On the left side of the photo above, Kathleen wears the wrong color blush. The bright red against her fair skin creates harsh angles. On the right, she's wearing a flattering peach.

Color, placement, and blending. I can't stress those words enough. If any one of those aspects of makeup application is out of sync, your face will be, too. That's especially true for blush.

Many women incorrectly try to use blush as a means of contouring the face, and that's when they get into trouble. The person who tries to "create" hollow cheeks or high cheekbones with blush inevitably ends up wearing too much. The result, typically, is a face that looks dirty—not a pretty picture. I'd rather see someone wearing no cheek color than too much. But, remember, this is the most common mistake women make.

As you can see in the photograph on the far left, improperly blended blush can be a disaster. In this case too much makeup was applied and no attempt was made to blend it. I always suggest that you apply blusher very lightly at first, to establish the best placement (see page 99). Intensify the color gradually, but use your blush brush to constantly blend so there's no war-paint line. You may want to reserve one brush just for blending. If you apply too much, use a sponge moistened with toner (not water, which can cause bacteria to grow) to absorb the excess color and a clean, dry sponge to reblend. If you remove too much, add back some color with the blush brush. Make sure the final effect is subtle and natural.

Follow the directions on page 99 carefully. Finding the bottom of your cheekbone is the only exacting way I know to determine the proper placement of your blush. When blush is placed too high or too low on the face, its benefits are lost. When it's too high, angles aren't defined or created. Instead, the area surrounding the eye is diminished, so the eye looks smaller and the undereye region looks puffy. Lines and creases around the eyes are accentuated when blush collects in the creases. Placed too low, blush drags the face down, making it look older and saggy.

Selecting the right color of blush is a straightforward procedure. When you go to a cosmetics counter you'll find dozens of shades of blusher and ten of them may be right for you—that's the fun of makeup. So pick a shade that you like.

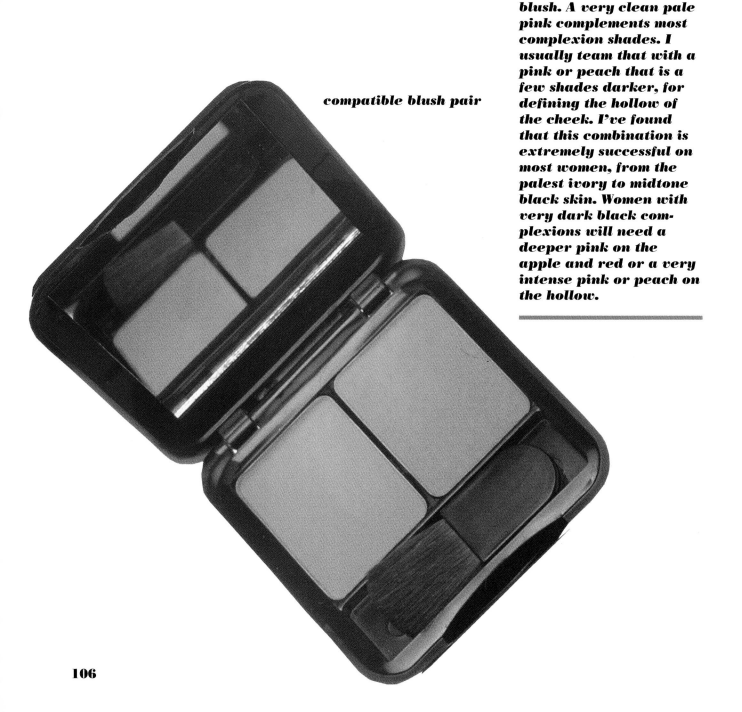

compatible blush pair

Remember, you need two shades to create the most natural-looking blush. A very clean pale pink complements most complexion shades. I usually team that with a pink or peach that is a few shades darker, for defining the hollow of the cheek. I've found that this combination is extremely successful on most women, from the palest ivory to midtone black skin. Women with very dark black complexions will need a deeper pink on the apple and red or a very intense pink or peach on the hollow.

Before you buy a blush in a store, apply the sample, take a mirror, and check the color outside in natural light. If you see that your cheeks are as noticeable as your eyes, the blush is too dark. If you see that the blush is lighter than your foundation, it's too light.

I'm not of the school that says blush must be in the same color family as lip and eye color. For all but the darkest complexions, I've found that pink blush is compatible with most eye makeup and lipstick. Don't be afraid to wear it with peaches, corals, fuchsia, berry, and any of the brown-toned neutrals. Peach is another good choice. However, if the peach has too much brown in it, it won't work with blue-red or blue-pink lipstick and eye shadow. Red is a good choice for evening, but apply sparingly and blend carefully. Many women with dark complexions will find that if pink blushes are too light, red is their best blush choice. For all complexion types, I avoid vivid fuchsia- and berry-toned blushes because they look too harsh. Blush is supposed to make you look like you when you're blushing. Who blushes fuchsia? Stick with your favorite pink, peach, or red.

Always keep in mind that cheek color must seem natural. When you blend with a brush or sponge, the color should fade away along the edges, leaving no lines of demarcation. I always prefer to use powder blush because, for me, it's the easiest to blend and achieves a very sheer finish. If you're not comfortable with powder, try the creams, gels, and color rubs on the market—the same guidelines about color, placement, and blending apply.

Tips for Selecting Blush

- Always try on blush—shades look different in the compact than they do on your cheeks.
- Never wear a blush that's too light—it looks as artificial as a blush that's too dark.
- Stay away from vivid cheek color unless you desire a dramatic, evening look.
- Always buy two blush shades at once, a light and a dark, to be sure they blend well.
- Save frosted blushes for special occasions.

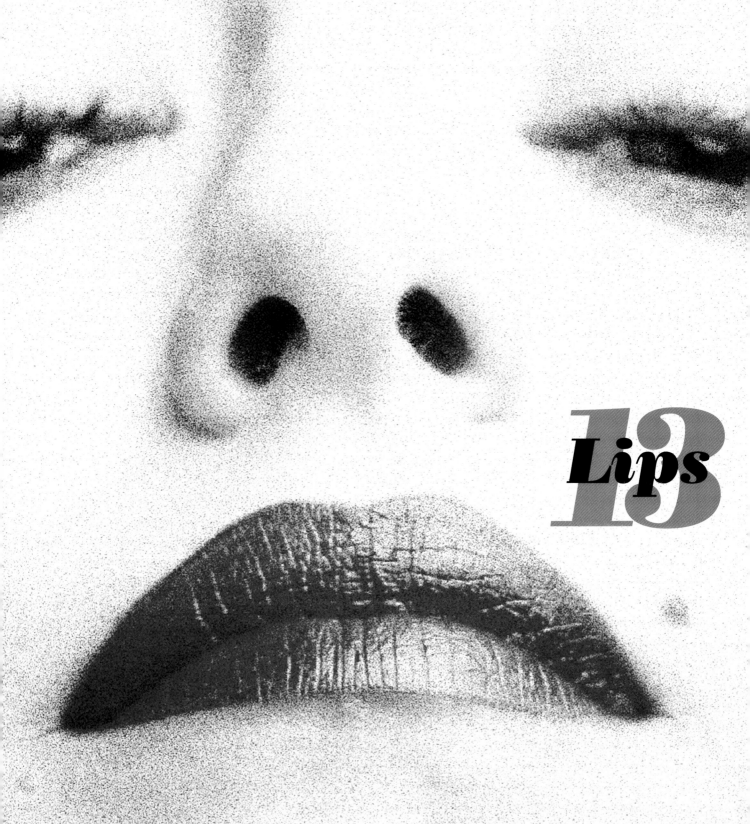

13 Lips

As I write this chapter, voluptuous mouths are in style. Women with average or thin lips are spending money to have them artificially plumped by cosmetic surgeons and dermatologists. Others are heading to tattoo artists to have permanent lines drawn outside the natural contours of their lips. Still others are loading on lip liners, lipstick, and gloss, trying desperately to create a succulent mouth.

Unfortunately, few of the results are good. Often the women's faces look terribly fake, and in the worst cases, their mouths are being permanently disfigured and their money is wasted, all for fashion's sake. I hate to think what happens next year (or even before this book goes to press) when the delicate, demure mouth is suddenly "in."

In this chapter you'll see mouths that look wonderful, yet no two pairs of lips are alike. They belong to women who aren't faking anything—they're enhancing what they've got.

I know your mouth looks beautiful, too. I encourage you to love your lips just the way they are. Then, show them off.

Lipstick color is a form of self-expression. That's why I've always suggested that women blend their own lipsticks. For that reason, when I sell lipstick I combine four shades in the same compact. Those are shown on the next page, not because I want you to run out and purchase my lipsticks (it would be nice!), but because it's an easy way for you to see what four-color palettes I recommend. The families of colors I show work well together. You may have similar shades in your cosmetics drawer right now. For the most variety, I suggest that you eventually build a lipstick wardrobe that includes three or four shades of red, pink, and peach. In each group, one shade should have a brownish cast, one bluish, one neutral. If you like a matte finish, add a neutral matte lipstick.

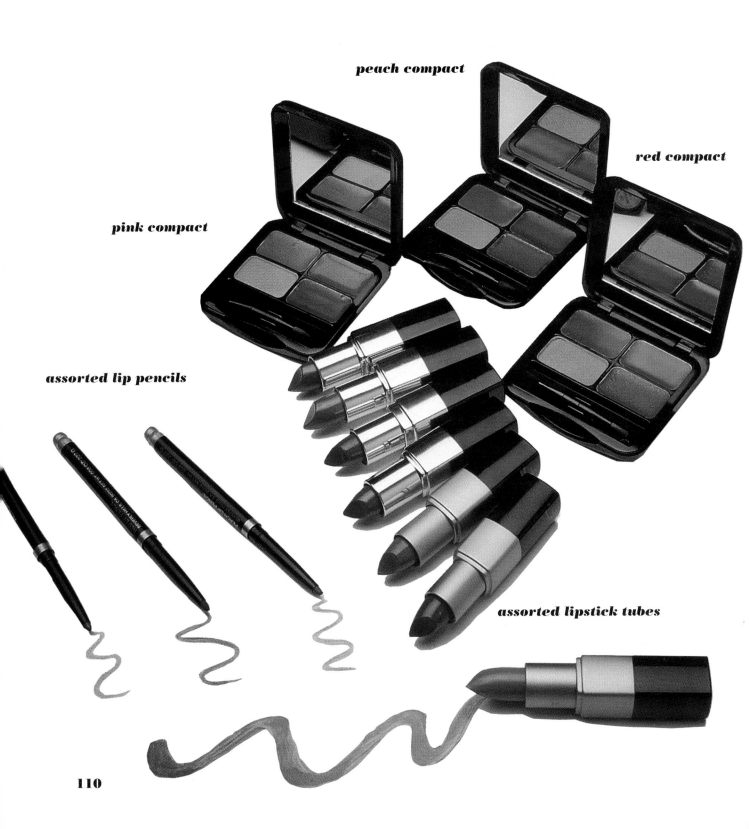

peach compact

red compact

pink compact

assorted lip pencils

assorted lipstick tubes

110

Group the shades as I have. Use a lip brush to blend them for an unlimited number of lipstick shades within a color family. You'll have enough variety to see yourself through all occasions, any time of day. One liner pencil should coordinate with each color group. You should also have one liner pencil that exactly matches your lips. Whether you choose tube or compact lip color, I find this to be the easiest and most economical way to purchase lipstick and liner.

I've heard many women say they can't wear red lipstick. I don't agree. In fact, I believe that every woman can wear any color of lipstick, as long as the shade is right. Some women look better in a blue red, others in a brownish red or orange red. It takes some experimentation to find the right shade, but that's the benefit (and fun) of blending your own.

Tips for Selecting Lip Color

- If your complexion is sallow, bright shades with a bluish cast will add a glow to your skin tone. If you prefer a more neutral lip, opt for brownish shades. Stay away from true orange shades, which tend to make your skin look more yellow.

- If your complexion has a ruddy cast, shades with a peach or brown cast work best for you.

- If your complexion is very fair, shades with a bluish cast work well on you.

- If your teeth are very yellow (this happens naturally as we age), avoid very bluish lipsticks, which tend to make them look more yellow.

- If you're still confused, play it safe and wear a shade that is close to the natural tone of your lips.

I added lipstick in tubes to my line because so many women requested them, but to tell the truth, the four-color lip compacts still outsell the tubes. I think that's because women have experienced how easy it is to blend custom colors and they appreciate that one compact means always having the right color in hand. No matter which form you choose, for the longest lasting results, always line the lips and then apply the color as shown in the steps on page 112.

Lipstick Application

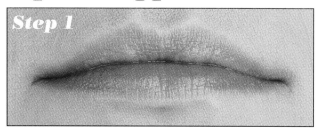

Step 1

Start with clean, dry lips. If lipstick wears off quickly, cover lips with foundation. If lips tend to be dry and cracked, use a lip conditioner first.

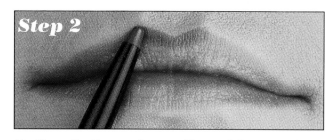

Step 2

Define the bow of your lips with your lip liner pencil.

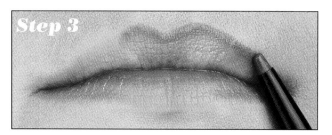

Step 3

Complete the line on each side of bow. Start at the top of bow and work toward outer corners.

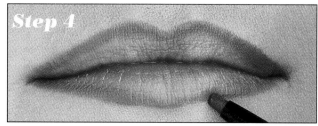

Step 4

Line lower lip with pencil.

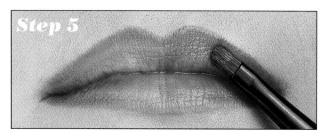

Step 5

Fill in upper lip with color using lipstick brush.

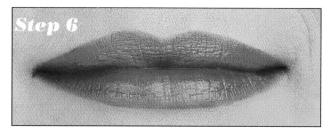

Step 6

Fill in lower lip with color using lipstick brush. Blot with a tissue. For longer-lasting results, color entire lip with lip pencil, apply lip color with brush, and blot.

30 Seconds to Beautiful Lips

It takes me 30 seconds or less to apply my lipstick, even though I use a lip pencil and blend my own colors with a lipstick brush. It may be a 10-second process straight from the tube, but you won't get the same precision. Try my method and you'll find it's worth the few extra seconds.

Lining with a lip pencil serves several purposes, the most important of which is to keep your lipstick in place. Lip liner also defines the unique shape of your lips. In addition, with lip pencil you can achieve special effects, such as maximizing or minimizing the size of your lips, without looking artificial. Sometimes for very long-lasting lip color, I cover my lips with lip pencil and add a coat of a nonwaxy lip conditioner. The effect is that of a natural-looking stain.

If you prefer to apply your lipstick straight from a tube rather than using a brush, don't neglect lining your lips with pencil, especially if the color tends to bleed into lines around the lips. Pencil will act as a waxy barrier that stops the lipstick from bleeding into crevices.

Tips for Lining Lips

- If your hand is unsteady when applying lip pencil, use the fine edge of your foundation sponge dipped in a bit of foundation to smooth the line. Move the sponge smoothly along the lip line.

- To define the bow of your lips, line the "V" with a lighter shade of pencil than used to outline the rest.

- For a pouty look, apply lip color, then add a lighter shade in the center of both lips.

- If your lips are naturally uneven in tone, cover with foundation first, then proceed with application steps.

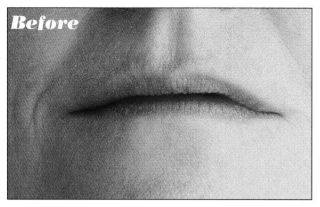

Before

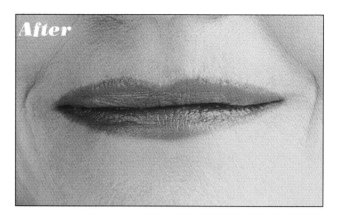

After

Thin Lips

Jaclyn has delicate lips that suit the other fine features on her face perfectly. The secret to beautiful thin lips is to color them completely, without overexaggerating them.

Here Jaclyn's lips are lined at the outside edge of the ridge on her lips, then the color is filled in. Her mouth looks naturally fuller. A coat of nonwaxy lip conditioner amplifies the color and keeps her lips soft.

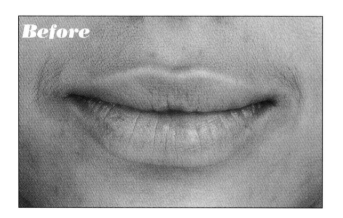

Before

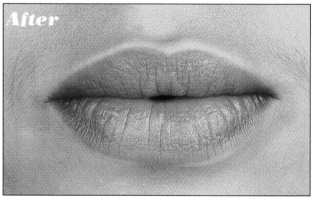

After

Full Lips

Wendy's lips are very full and have a beautiful shape. She can approach color two ways: to the outside edge of the ridge for maximum fullness, or to the inside edge of ridge to minimize.

Here Wendy's lips look a bit slimmer, and the natural ridge serves as a beautiful frame for her mouth. The secret is to follow the natural contours of the lips, inside the ridge.

Minor Adjustments

Since lips and eyes are the two most expressive features on the face, you naturally want them to look their best. The section on eye makeup demonstrated how different types of eyes can be enhanced with makeup, and the same can be done with your lips. No matter what their size or shape, most lips are extremely attractive. The way you use your mouth to speak, to smile, to show other emotions (let's not forget kissing!) all add to its distinctive beauty.

Few people would remember your mouth as anything but beautiful. That's because unless your mouth is very pretty, others focus on your eyes and don't notice your lips. If your mouth is particularly beautiful, you should emphasize it. And if you feel that it's not as striking as your eyes, make up your mouth to be naturally pretty, but not to be the focal point of your face. If you are dissatisfied with the shape or size of your lips, you can make minor yet effective adjustments with color.

I never encourage anyone to dramatically change the look of their lips with makeup. Although recontouring with cosmetic tricks can do startling things in still photographs, it never looks as natural in person. But makeup can be a tool to enhance the natural shape and size of the lips. Everyone's mouth is defined by a ridge around the perimeter of the rosy pigment of the lips. Use this ridge to very naturally determine the placement of your lip color. To minimize the look of the lips, line the inner edge of the ridge with pencil and apply lipstick just to the liner. To make them look fuller, line the outer edge of the ridge and extend lipstick over the ridge to the liner. Frosted lipsticks and pale lipsticks tend to make the lips look fuller, while a matte finish and subdued colors deemphasize natural fullness.

Lip pencil can also be used to balance uneven lips, add a bit of shape to lips that lack a bow, and help solve some of the problems that occur as lips age. On the next few pages are examples of minor adjustments that make a major difference.

Minor Adjustments

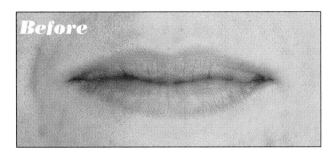

Before

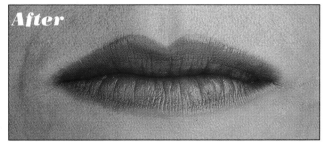

After

Small Mouth

Laura's mouth is small in proportion to her face, but her lips have a beautiful shape that can look very dramatic with the right lip color.

Laura's lips look their fullest when she uses lip pencil on the outside edge of the lip ridge all the way to the outside corners of the mouth. A nonwaxy lip conditioner adds some additional shine for a fuller look.

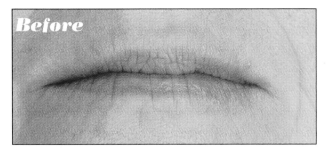

Before

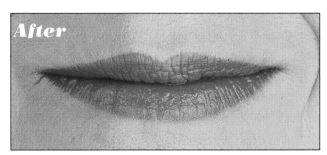

After

Undefined Lips

Despite their even proportions, Gloria's lips don't have the shape or fullness that she wants. She can strengthen them easily with color and adjust the shape by a fraction.

Covering the center of her upper lip with foundation and drawing a short, wide "V" in the center gives Gloria a bow. From top of the "V," she extends lines to the corners, rounding the curve of the bow. She lines the outside edge of the lip ridge on her lower lip, fills in with color, and adds a lighter shade in the center of her lips for highlight.

116

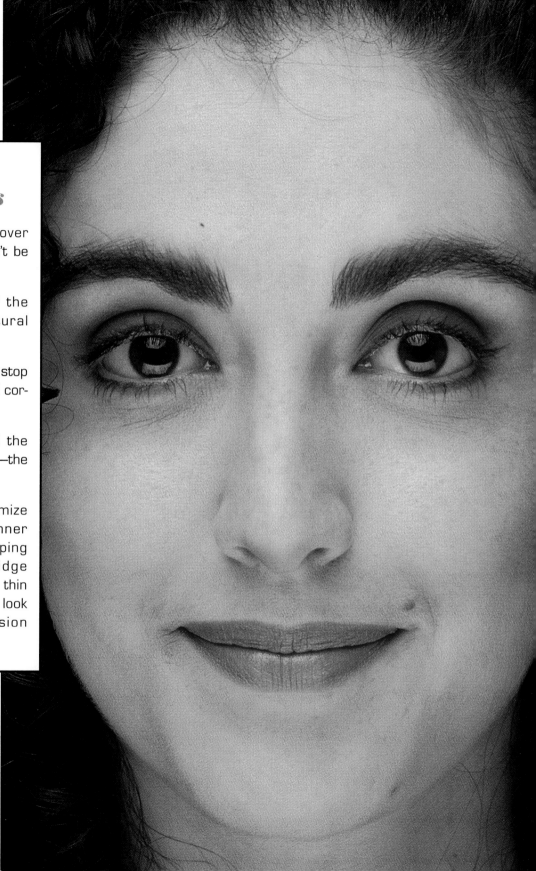

Tips for Minor Adjustments

• Use foundation to cover natural pigment if it won't be covered completely.

• Round the peaks of the bow for the most natural look.

• To shorten wide lips, stop lip liner inside the natural corners.

• Never outline beyond the natural ridge of the lips—the result looks clownish.

• When trying to minimize the lips, line on the inner ridge of the lips. Stopping short of that inner ridge makes the lips look too thin and shapeless—the lips look older and the expression looks angry.

More Minor Adjustments

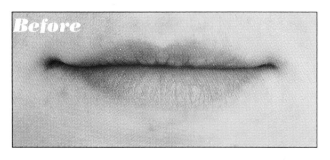

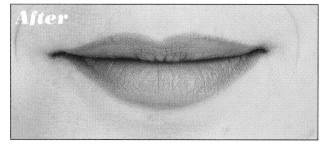

Unbalanced Lips

Gabrielle's upper lip is much thinner than her lower lip, creating the look of a constant pout. Though this is charming, she can balance her lips with lip pencil if she wants.

By using liner on the outside edge of the ridge of her upper lip only and following the natural contours of her lower lip, Gabrielle has adjusted the shape of her mouth, which now appears to be in balance. A slightly lighter lipstick on the top lip also makes it look more prominent.

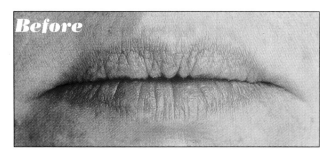

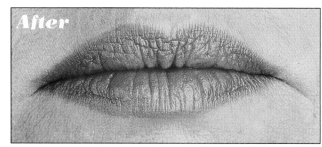

Downturned Mouth

The corners of Elizabeth's mouth turn down a bit. She can create a happier look with a slight adjustment at the corners of the upper lip.

Rather than following the natural lip line at the corners, Elizabeth extends the line of the upper lip slightly above the natural corner, creating a "<" and ">" on the skin. Then she fills in the lip color, and highlights the center of the lips with a light shade to focus attention there.

Typical Lip Lining Mistakes

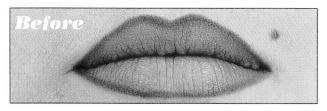

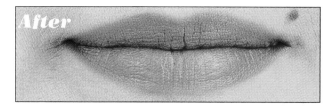

Too Much Liner

When the lip liner is too dark, the entire lip makeup looks wrong. There's nothing natural-looking about this mouth.

Lip pencil should be subtle, so there's no demarcation between liner and lipstick color, yet the edge is neatly defined.

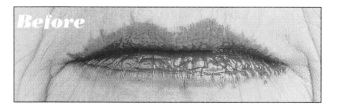

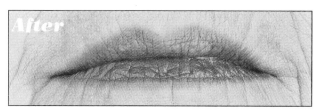

Bleeding Lipstick

Trish's lips have age lines, but they haven't diminished the beautiful shape of her lips. Her "supermoist" lipstick bleeds into the crevices and accentuates fine wrinkles.

By lining the lips with pencil and using a matte lipstick, Trish reduces the chances of the color seeping into the crevices. Avoid lip glosses and "supermoist" lipsticks.

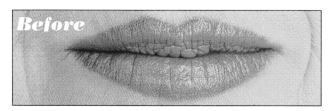

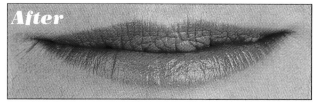

Overcorrected Lips

These lips were overcorrected—the change is too obvious. The lip liner is drawn directly on the skin, beyond the outside edge of the lips.

Here the line follows the outside edge of the ridge, and a bit of extra foundation is used as a highlight on the bow to make the lips look fuller.

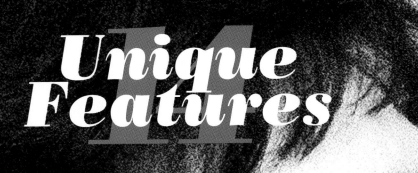

Unique
Features
14

This was the most difficult chapter for me. At first I had called it "special problems," and I couldn't figure out why no ideas were coming to me. I soon realized it's because I never look at a face and see a "problem." Yet since women write and call me, concerned about "problems"—wide noses, pointed chins, broad foreheads, and the like—I got caught in the negative-word trap. Once I turned it around and realized what my topic actually is, it was easy to get started. See how debilitating negative thinking can be?

First of all, there's nothing inherently "wrong" with your face; you have no "problem" features. I want you to believe me when I say that. Your face is a special composition of each of your unique characteristics. Would we look at old photos of Marilyn Monroe and say that her chin was too broad, or do we call Liz Taylor's too sharp? Is Paulina Porizkova's nose too thin and Cindy Crawford's mole too dark? I never look at a face and want to change it. My approach is to play up everything that's beautiful, which in turn enhances the entire face.

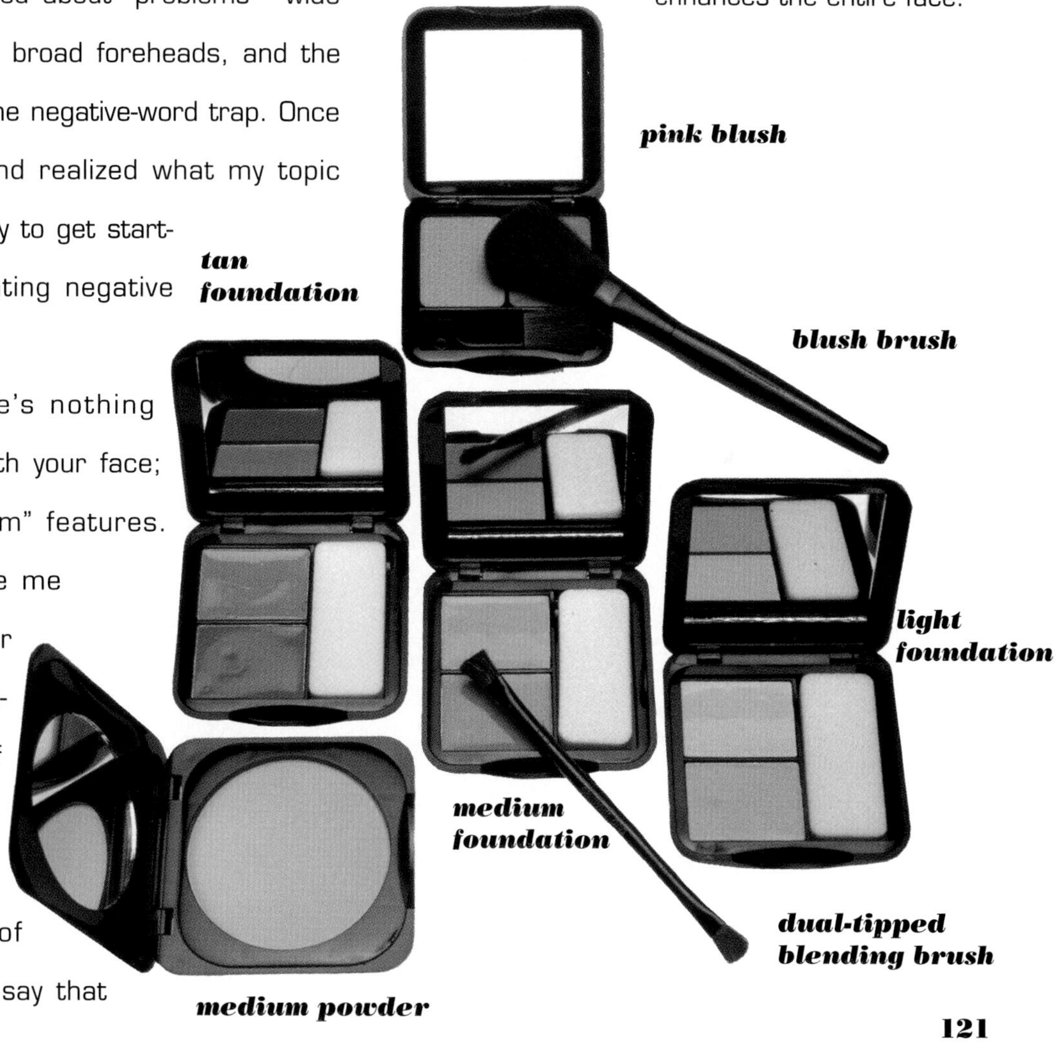

pink blush

tan foundation

blush brush

light foundation

medium foundation

dual-tipped blending brush

medium powder

121

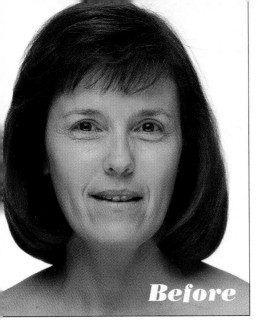

Before

Undefined Cheekbones

Kathleen occasionally likes a dramatic, high-cheekbone look. Although the shape of her face is very attractive without any contouring makeup, she can achieve considerably more definition by playing with shadow and highlight. Using a Q-Tip swab, apply a line of dark foundation under cheekbone from ear toward nose. Blend line until blurred, creating a shadow under cheekbone. Shadow should be most intense in the hollow. Highlight cheekbone itself with a bit of lighter foundation. Now add blush as indicated on page 99.

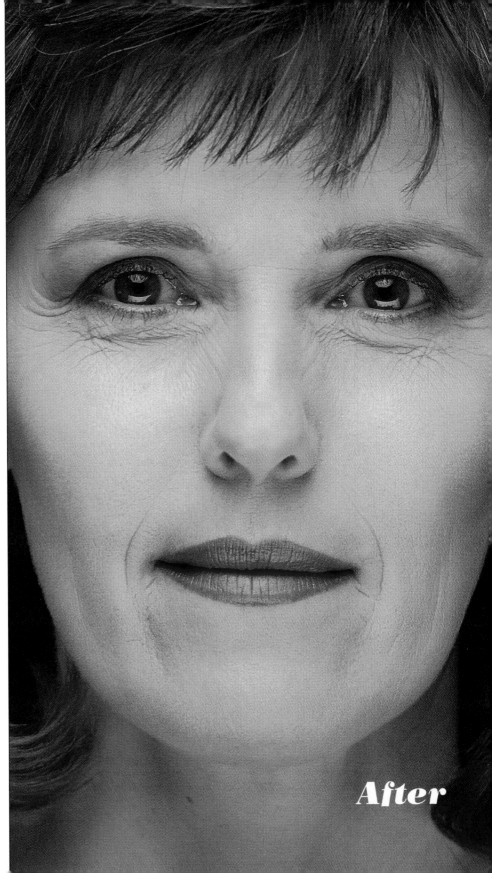

After

On the other hand, I never discourage anyone from using "corrective" makeup if there's something about her face that bugs her and she can minimize it with a little makeup trick. That's what makeup artists do all the time, especially when preparing someone for a photograph. I wouldn't recommend using these techniques every day—it's too much of a bother. But they work, so use them when you want a little lift.

The process depends on shadow and highlight. Shadows will create the illusion of slimming an area and highlight will broaden it. I create shadows by using a foundation one shade darker than that used on the rest of the face. Highlights are achieved, as I mentioned in the foundation chap-

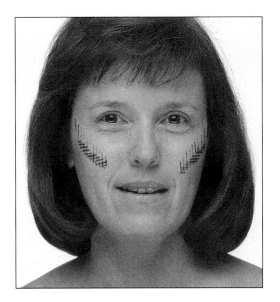

ter, with base one shade lighter than usual. Any darker or lighter than one shade in either direction will become too difficult to blend, so you won't be pleased with the results. With only a slight variation in tone you'll notice the difference when you look in the mirror, but you probably won't feel like you're wearing a lot of makeup.

As I've stressed in so many places throughout this makeup section, blending is of foremost importance. If you felt your nose was too obvious because it was wide, it will be considerably more obvious with discernible stripes of light and dark foundation. Contouring techniques are effective only if they're well executed. So be certain to blend with a blush brush or with your fingertips until each shade fades into the other.

In the black-and-white photo on the left and on the following pages, the crosshatching indicates where to place shading and highlighter.

Pointed Chin

Kristen's strong, pointed chin adds a delightful angle to her otherwise round face and gives her lots of personality. This very defined area of her face also draws attention to her beautiful full lips. But many women with prominent chins look in the mirror and don't see anything else. I urge them to recognize the chin as the V that focuses attention on the mouth and eyes. Enhancing lips and eyes often eliminates the need to minimize the chin. To soften a pointed chin, blend dark foundation on the tip; blend so it fades under the jawline. Use the lightest foundation on either side of the darker shading. Blend and powder.

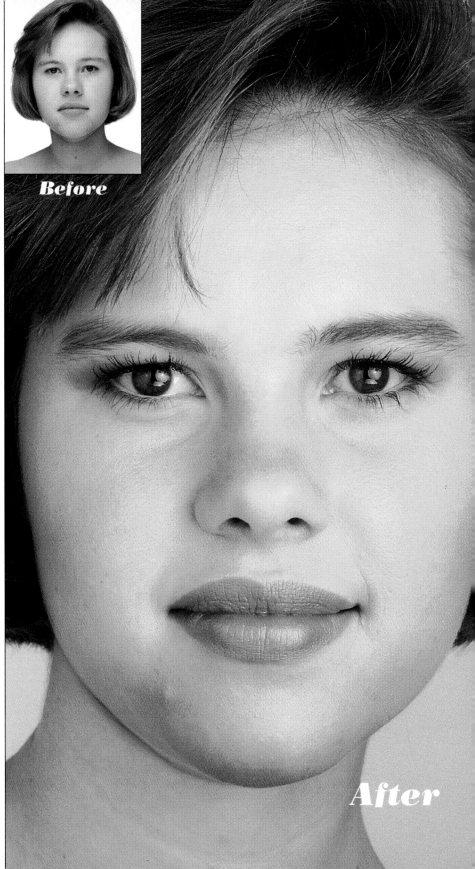

Before

After

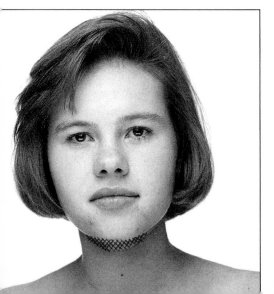

Undefined Chin

Like so many women over 35, Roberta notices her soft chin line more than other people do. Naturally when she's in a photograph labeled "Undefined Chin," our eyes zero in on it. Normally, extra fullness is obvious only when we tilt our chin down. A woman changes her look by improving her posture, remembering to hold the head high. For photographs and special occasions, contouring makeup provides extra insurance, however. With a Q-Tip draw a thick line of dark foundation along the jawbone. With a sponge, blur the line, blending down over the area of fullness. Call attention upward on the face with nice eye and cheek makeup.

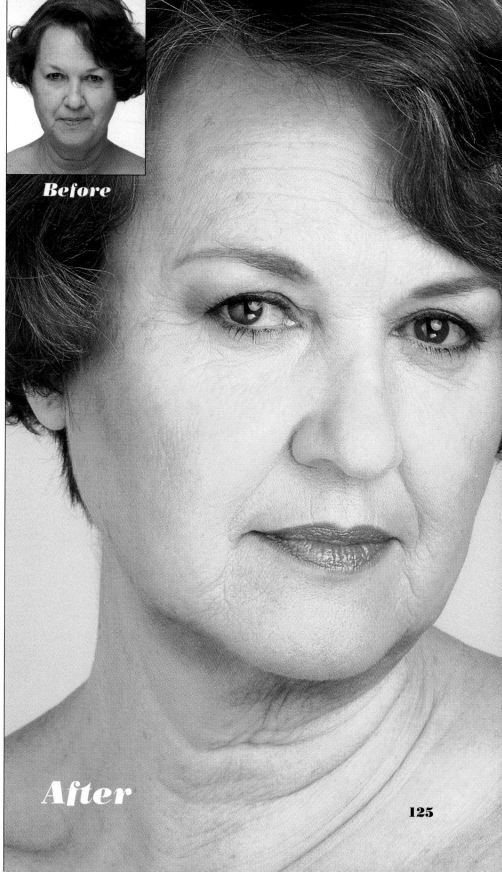

Before

After

125

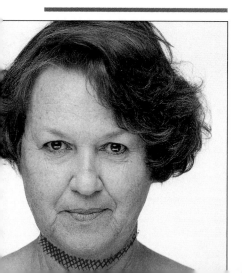

Broad Chin

Gloria's broad chin doesn't look like a "problem" to me—it gives her face a sophisticated shape. But many women prefer to look narrower in the jaw. A simple shading method creates a slimmer illusion. The same technique can be used to camouflage a sagging jawline. Before using the contouring tricks, however, call attention to the lips, cheeks, and eyes, and the wide or sagging jaw may seem insignificant. To slim the area with makeup, use a Q-Tip or sponge with dark foundation to shade the jawbone from the center of the chin up toward the ear. Blend carefully. Add light foundation as highlight at center of chin. Blend.

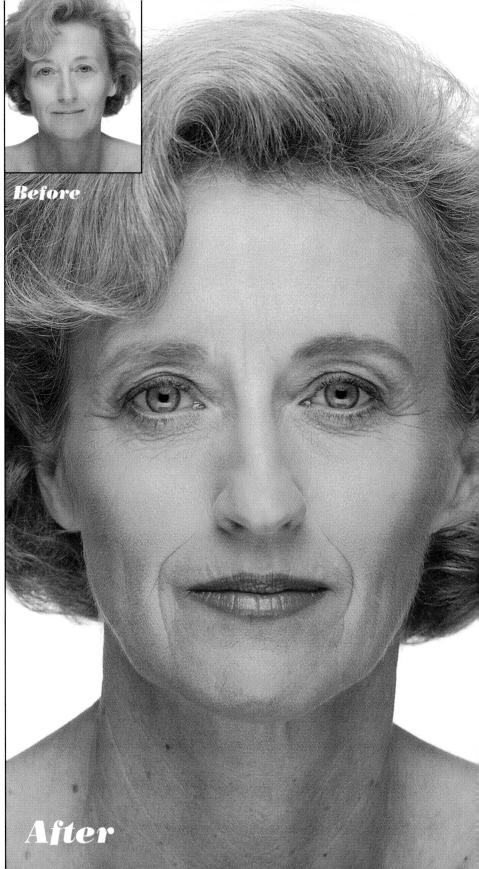

Before

After

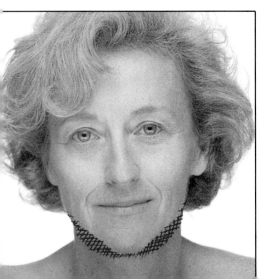

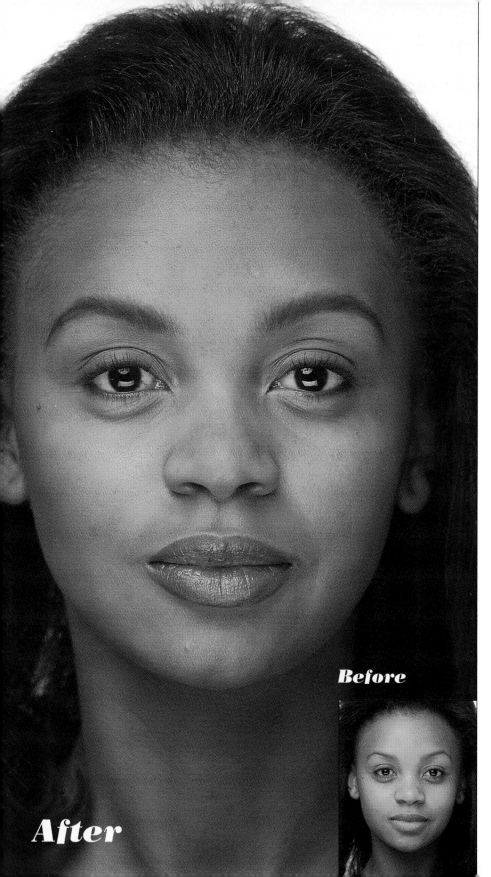

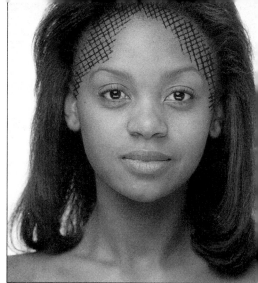

Wide Forehead

Camey's wide forehead gives her face a beautiful heart shape, so she plays it up by brushing her hair back off her face. Notice that her forehead offsets her eyes very dramatically, and the arch of her brow emphasizes the elegant width at the top of her head. Some women would rather minimize their wide foreheads. The first step would be to add bangs or soft waves at the temples. But a little contouring is easy to do. Use a makeup sponge to add dark foundation to the temples and above the outer half of the brows. Blend carefully. Dust light blush in the center of the forehead as a highlight.

Before

After

127

Wide Nose

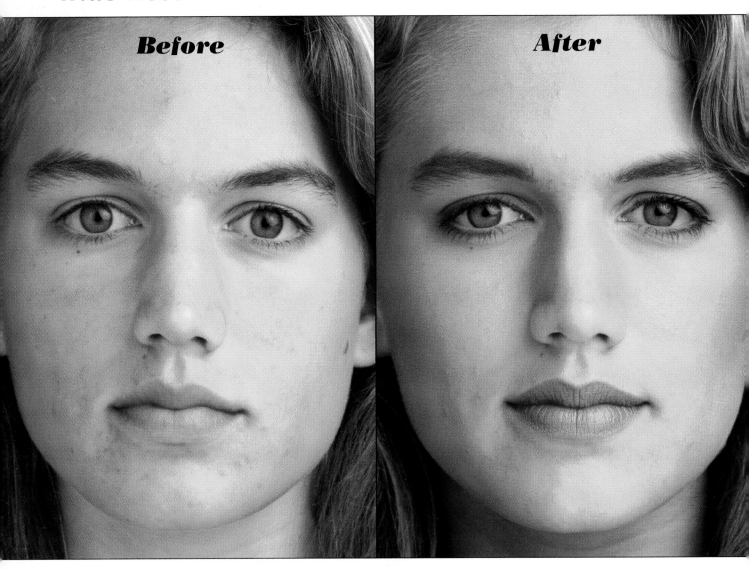

Before

After

Lisa's wide nose is certainly not a drawback. It suits the proportion of her face. However, if its width bothers her, she can alter the illusion with light and dark makeup. With a wedge sponge or Q-Tip, apply a straight line of darker foundation to each side of the nose, from bridge to nostrils. Blend. Then, with a Q-Tip dipped in the lighter foundation, draw a line down the center of the nose as a highlight. Blend.

Long Nose/Bump on Nose

Paula has a pretty, graceful nose. But if she feels her nose is too long, she can do a quick trick with makeup. After applying a touch of dark foundation under the tip, blending the color around half of the nostrils will foreshorten the nose. Elizabeth's nose has a tiny bump near the bridge—it isn't necessary to try to cover it. But if a bump bothers you, it too can be minimized with makeup. Apply dark foundation directly on the raised area. Shade the sides of the nose from the bridge to the end, and use a Q-Tip to draw a line down the center of the nose from the bottom of the bump to the tip. Blend with a clean sponge.

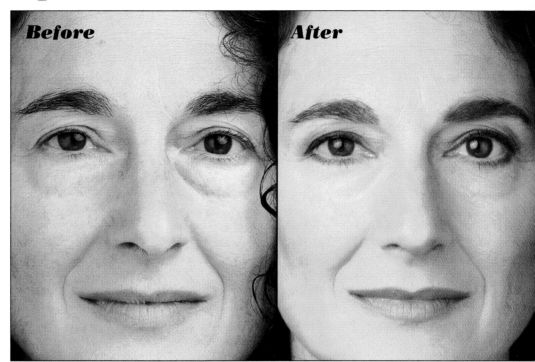

Before **After**

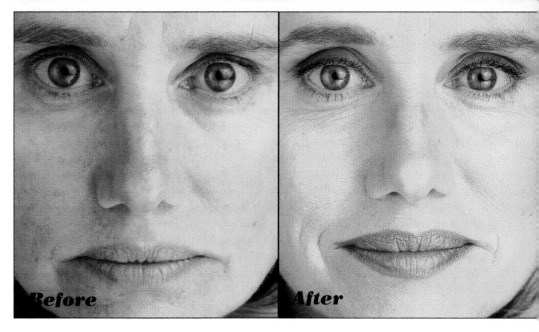

Before **After**

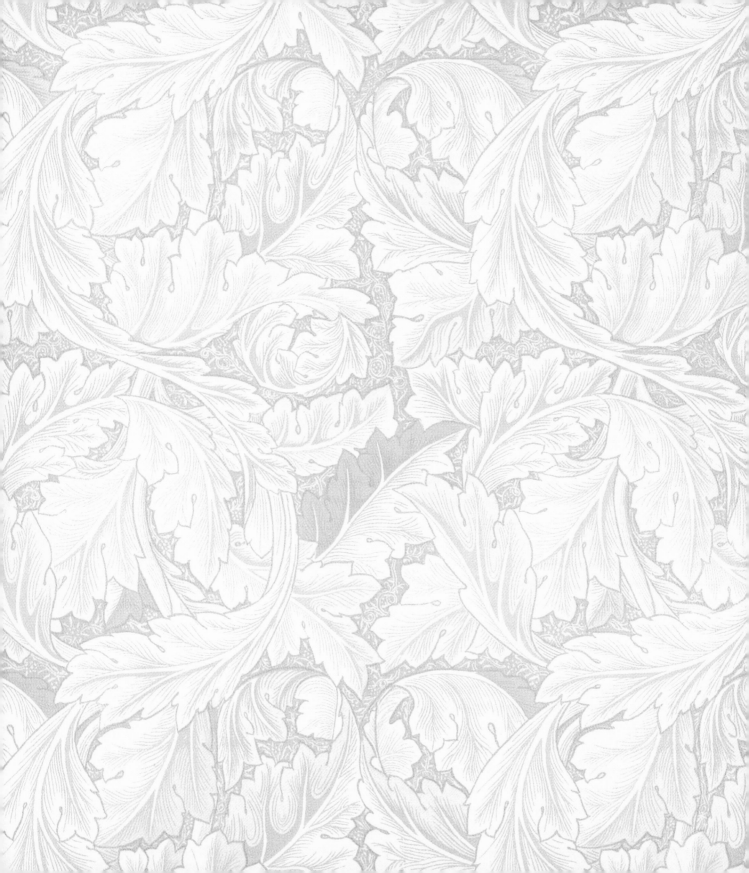

Personal Best

4

Remember, putting on a fresh, new makeup look is only a preliminary step toward feeling your personal best. When you start to make things happen in your life, your self-esteem will soar. In this final section, I'll share some success stories that I hope will inspire you as much as they've inspired me.

Role Models

We all need role models. As we work to achieve our personal best, these are the people whose images we admire, the people we'd most like to emulate in one way or another. They inspire us, help us to establish our individual goals, and provide guidance in an indirect or direct way.

Sometimes they can frustrate us, too, especially if we confuse idols with role models. Like most teenagers, when I was young I'd look through the pages of fashion magazines to pick out all the beautiful models I wanted to look like. Twiggy and the Yardley model Jean Shrimpton were my idols. To me, they were the greatest. My best friend—a gorgeous blue-eyed blonde, the prom queen, who fit every facet of the all-American girl—was another one of my role models. It didn't matter that I would never look like Twiggy (I wasn't rail thin and flat-chested), or Jean Shrimpton (I don't have a little nose and high cheekbones), or my best friend (my hair and eyes are dark brown). They, to me, were the measure of ideal beauty, and at the time, most people agreed with me. Of course, looking back, I realize that by establishing them as my touchstones, there was no room for me to be pretty. I would never look like them. I was setting myself up to feel inadequate at best and ugly at worst. I was forgetting to appreciate my own looks. I had confused idols for role models.

Fortunately I got through the teen years. As I mentioned in the introduction to this book, when I first started as a makeup artist, I spent several years continuing to compare myself to movie stars and models. As I gained more confidence in myself and my work, I lost the need to look like the celebrities, especially since I realized very quickly that most of them were no happier than I, just richer. The stars were asking me for beauty advice and for my products. Actually, when it dawned on me that I was more confident about my looks than many of them were about theirs, my self-esteem soared. That's when I realized that my knowledge was worthwhile and would be of help to many women in many fields.

That's also when my role models became more appropriate. Estee Lauder was one; Beverly Sassoon was another. Mrs. Lauder had, of course, achieved the ultimate in cosmetics success: a multibillion-dollar cosmetics empire, a happy family, the respect of the world. Beverly, who was a friend and already had developed a makeup line (albeit on a much smaller scale than Mrs. Lauder's) at the time I was developing mine, was, for me, the perfect image of a cosmetics company executive. She was not only smart and successful, but perfectly groomed and stylishly dressed. "She's got the whole look," I used to tell myself, noting that she had played up all the positives of her face with makeup and always had a positive attitude. I started visualizing myself succeeding in the many different ways these women had.

As my company began to grow, so did my self-confidence; soon I wasn't trying to be like anyone else in my profession. Because I was one of the pioneers in televised cosmetics sales, old marketing methods had become irrelevant to my business. Charting a new course became a constant challenge. I was excited about my own achievements, my own success. Now when I speak at colleges and young women tell me that I'm their role model, I'm reminded of how important selecting appropriate role models was to me.

> **EXERCISE:** Make two lists. On list 1, write the names of the women you respect most. On list 2, name the women you think are most beautiful. List the reasons you put each woman on each list. Which list is longer? Which list is the most specific? Chances are you answer list 1 to both questions. Now think of the faces of the women on list 1 and analyze them—what positive qualities do they possess? Which list holds the names of the women you feel are your role models or are worthy of being your role models? On which list would you rather be?

These days, the spectrum of women I admire has broadened tremendously. Diane Sawyer, Gloria Steinem, and Oprah Winfrey inspire me now—women who are involved and accomplished. They have their own ideas and are committed to what they believe in. These women proceed with a strong sense of self.

On the personal side, my mother is always on my list, and so is my sister, a psychologist in the Los Angeles County prison system. And, of course, there's my friend Ali MacGraw.

Ali has contagious enthusiasm—about everything. After five minutes with her, I'm energized and excited. She's always brimming with ideas. She doesn't take anything for granted—not her great looks, her career, or her personal life.

Having lived through as many ups and downs as the rest of us, she knows that self-esteem is a precious commodity that has to be nurtured. "When I'm feeling down about myself, I meditate to try to figure out what's wrong and to get centered," she once told me. "Then I go to the gym and run some oxygen through my ego. I feel the best mentally when I'm feeling good physically." Despite how beautiful she is, she hasn't allowed her self-esteem to be determined by her appearance.

"If I don't like myself, no amount of applause is going to convince me that I'm okay," she told me one day when we were sipping tea in a Brentwood deli. "That's on a Hollywood level, but it's the same in the real world, too. I've noticed that when I feel centered and calm, people say I look great. When I'm not feeling that way, they don't. Makes perfect sense, doesn't it? I don't think most human beings can separate the way they're feeling inside from the way they look—at least not for long. And painting on a totally foreign face is not going to change anything."

When I talk to Ali, it's clear to me that her beauty comes from her inner strength, not vice versa. Her appearance clinched the first modeling jobs, which initially led to the movie roles in Hollywood, but her talent, determination, and intelligence made her a success.

Some of my newest role models came to my attention because they wrote to tell me about their personal successes when I sponsored a life-style makeover contest a few years ago. I am constantly impressed with the ways in which so many women have taken charge of their lives and accomplished exactly what they set out to do...and more. Four of these remarkable women have shared their stories with me. They've met incredible challenges, each in very different ways. I want you to meet each of them—you'll be inspired by their successes. (And for a bit more inspiration, their photos will show you how great these women look with or without makeup.)

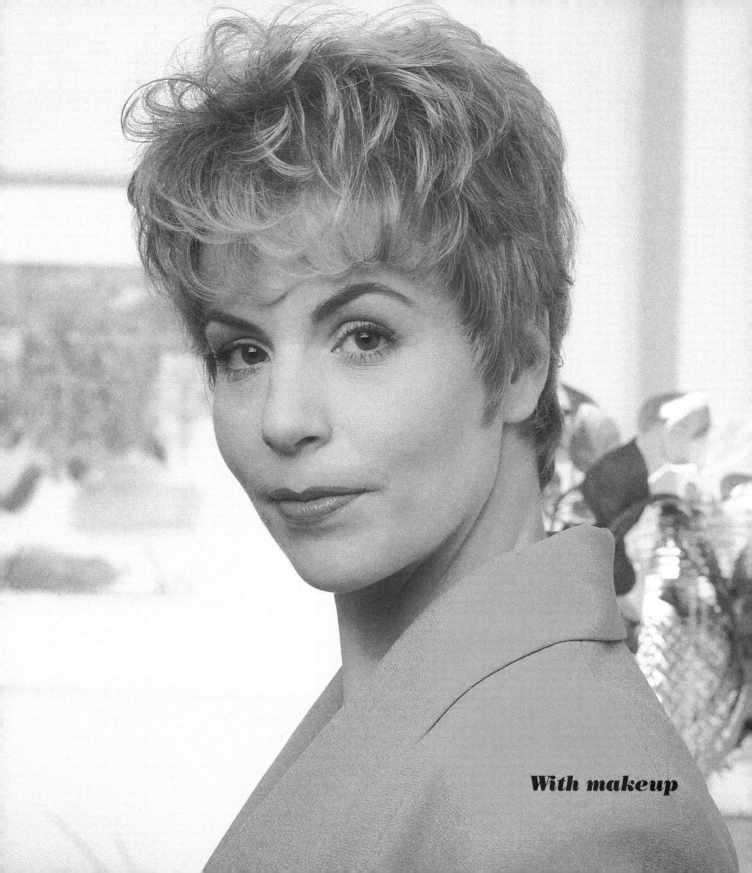

With makeup

Lorraine Kacanich

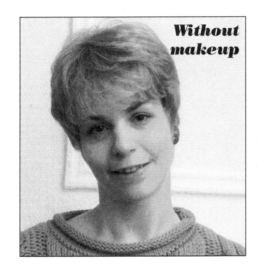

Without makeup

In the summer of 1988, Lorraine Kacanich had a life worth celebrating. Happily married five years, she had two beautiful children. After much discussion, she and her husband had decided they were financially able, so Lorraine elected to take a break from her career in the publishing industry to stay home as a full-time mom.

Though she felt fortunate and happy, on one hand, to be able to devote her life to her children, another part of her missed the intellectual challenge and social interaction that the workplace provides. Then her husband's union went on strike, he was out of work for seventeen weeks, they had no health care coverage—times were difficult. In those stressful times, Lorraine found solace in food.

"I was on the verge of my thirtieth birthday and my weight had blossomed (or more accurately 'ballooned') to an unbelievable 230 pounds—I'm only five three!" she recalls. Instead of the fitted business suits she had worn to work, her day-in, day-out wardrobe consisted of sweatpants and sweatshirts.

"At that stage, losing weight seemed impossible to me—I was 80 pounds heavier than when I left work," Lorraine remembers. "I was disappointed in myself, and I had lost my self-confidence." The reactions from strangers affected her most deeply: "You're looked at differently when you're fat. People treat you disrespectfully. When you go into a store and need a size 22 dress, salespeople aren't always sympathetic."

Her self-esteem had dipped to its lowest when she finally realized that she was the only one who could change her life. "One day I was in the car and I caught a glimpse of myself in the side-view mirror—I was a mess. My hair wasn't done. No makeup. I didn't recognize myself. I decided that very minute that I was going to make some changes in my life."

Lorraine took action. She decided to go back to college to pursue her R.N. so she could contribute to the security of her family and increase her self-esteem. "Just making the decision to continue my education made me feel better. Then, when I started classes I felt that sense of challenge again."

But there were drawbacks. Since she was ten years older than most of the other students, "I'd sweat walking up the hill to class—I was out of shape, and I really noticed it when I compared myself to the other nursing students," she explains.

During her first year, she began to change her image, partly to compensate for her weight and partly, she acknowledges now, because she was gearing up for a complete change. She began wearing natural-looking makeup and maintaining her hair. She started receiving words of encouragement about her appearance from her classmates.

"I realized that your face is what you present to the world—if you look like you care, people respond differently," she says. "I was living proof. People were starting to tell me that I was pretty. It had been a long time since I'd heard those words. It helped build my confidence."

But that was just the beginning. Soon Lorraine was able to tackle her biggest problem. "Here I was, training to be a health professional, and I wasn't projecting a healthy image. I was carrying 80 extra pounds. I worried that my weight was going to get in the way of my career." Determined that she wouldn't undermine her own success, Lorraine went on a self-imposed diet that was nutritionally balanced. Within six months she had lost 85 pounds.

In her freshman year Lorraine's grades were so good that she won a navy scholarship to continue her studies. She went on to become president of her school's nursing association and is a member of the national honor society for her profession. Now a member of the U.S. Navy, she has earned her nursing cap and is working in military hospitals. She has applied to universities to complete her master's degree so she can become a family nurse practitioner.

Taking charge of her own life resulted in other plusses for Lorraine. "So many things have happened at home that let me know I made the right choice for my whole family. My husband, Gary, has decided that he wants to go back and continue his own education and my seven-year-old son wants to be a nurse. And that's not all—now Gary thinks in terms of the active things we can do together. He just bought a bicycle for me so we can ride together and we're planning to take a scuba class. Our life is more fun and active than it has ever been," relates a beaming Lorraine. She also credits her mother, who lives with the family, for her major support—she cares for the children while Lorraine and Gary work. "It's a team effort at our house—all based on love and trust," Lorraine says.

"Sometimes I pull out the pants I used to wear just to remind myself of what happens when you don't like yourself," Lorraine explains. "I'm at a weight that's healthy for me now, I'm working at a job I love, and I'm happy, really happy."

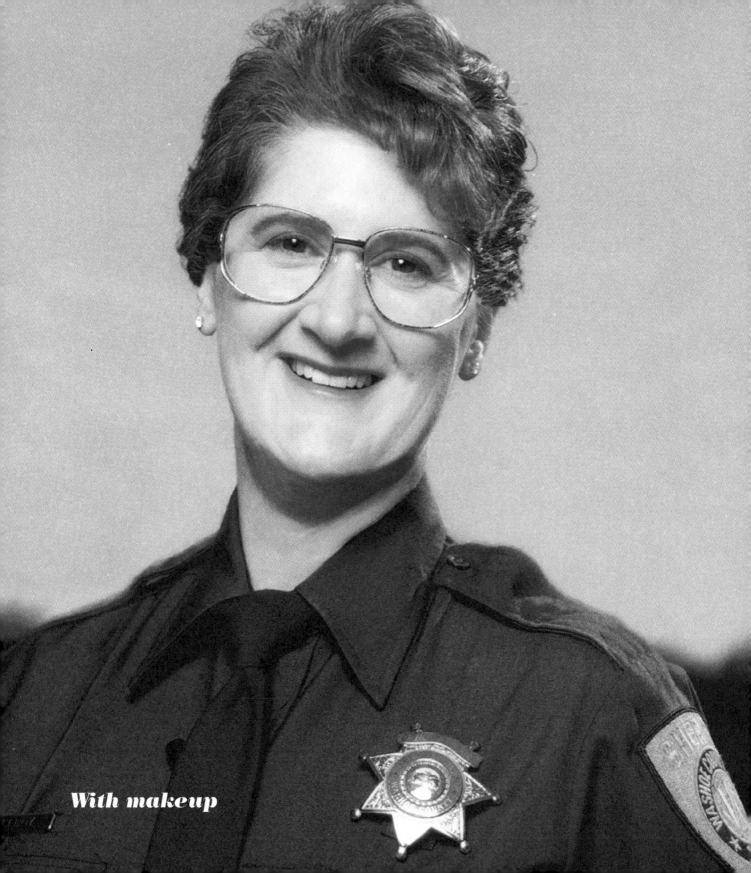

With makeup

Janice McElroy

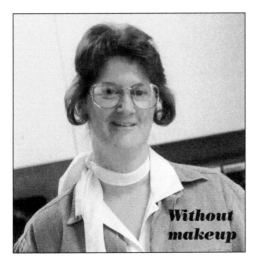

Without makeup

When she first wrote to me, Janice McElroy was a forty-one-year-old mother of three who had never held a full-time job outside the home. Raising her kids and running a bustling household had kept her too busy to devote eight hours a day to anything else. But with seemingly boundless energy, she held a few part-time jobs and took classes toward her college degree in computer science. Janice was well aware that one day she wanted another career in addition to being wife and mom.

One day, as she tells the story, "I decided that I had made enough beds. No more bus driver, dishwasher, and cook. I had to do something for me." But, frustrated by a lack of specific skills, Janice didn't know exactly how to start finding her place in the sun. Always a resourceful A student throughout school, she started researching. When an advertisement for a local job fair appeared in the local newspaper, she and a friend headed over to the site in hopes of inspiration. That the day would change her life hadn't occurred to her.

On a whim, with no thought of actually being qualified, Janice filled out a form for the job that appealed to her most: deputy sheriff. "I'd never held a gun, let alone thought about shooting one, and I'd never considered being a law enforcement officer. But I liked the idea of a career in a field that I could be proud of, so I put in my application."

Within a few weeks she was called in for a succession of qualifying tests: first a written exam; then the oral interview. She was one of the highest scorers and was one of three finalists out of the hundred who had passed the tests. Then came the intense personal scrutiny. The sheriff's departments gave her a polygraph test, drug and physical fitness tests, investigated her credit rating, screened her family members, contacted her acquaintances all over the country, checked her driver's record. Deemed the ideal candidate after three months of rigorous testing, Janice was offered the job. Three weeks later she was in training.

During that testing period Janice determined that a polished image was going to help her chances of success, but she learned that giving herself some confidence about her appearance had other ramifications. "I was nervous and knew that I needed everything working on my side. I dressed up for every interview, and always wore appropriate makeup. Prior to that I had never been a true makeup user. But once I found the right products I was encouraged. Looking good made me feel good. Pretty soon I wanted to go farther. I joined a gym to work with weights, tried to watch my diet, and promised to do something just for fun once a week." Now she takes martial arts classes and jogs in addition to her weight training to keep in shape, a must for a job that demands superb physical condition.

I remember so clearly that she ended her letter this way:

"I refuse to give up. If I can find a makeup that works for me, I can do anything. —a future Deputy Sheriff, Janice McElroy."

I was impressed with her determination then. Now that I've learned what she does in that position, I'm even more impressed. Today Janice is a full-fledged deputy working in an innovative prison facility in Washoe County, Nevada. The direct supervisor of more than seventy male inmates, five-foot-two-inch Janice carries no gun (although she has developed her skill and is now an accomplished marksman), but rather depends on her highly trained skills in interpersonal communication to keep the prisoners in line. Being female in a predominantly male environment is a decided challenge.

"When I first started, some of the other female deputies told me not to wear makeup or perfume because the men couldn't handle it. They urged me to look like a man. I followed their advice for a while, but I didn't feel right about it. I knew that my job was to earn respect for me. The real me wears makeup and a nice clean fragrance, so I went back to wearing both on the job. I act professional, look professional, and I'm gaining respect. That's the way I'm most comfortable."

Janice is thrilled with her new life, and so is her family. And by the way, her twenty-three-year-old son and his wife just had a baby daughter. She delights in the double challenge—"Now I'm learning to be a new grandma and a new deputy."

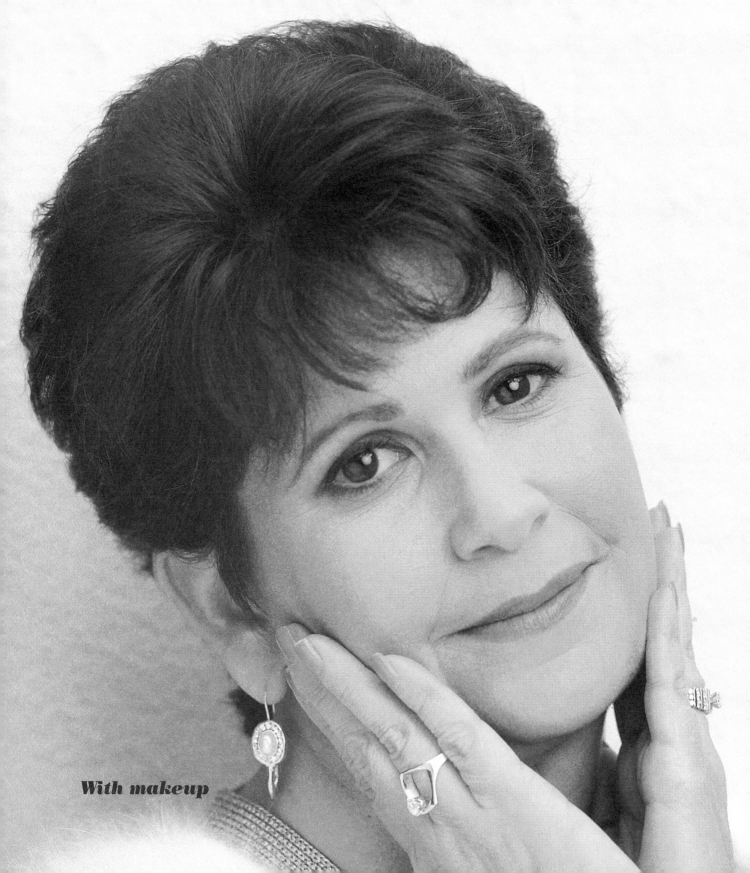

With makeup

Vinni Parrinello

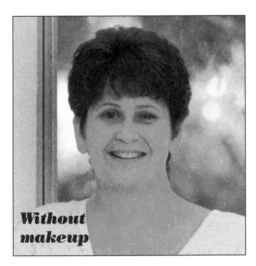

Without makeup

Talk about a tale of courage. Vinni Parrinello shared a remarkable story of the determination to live despite the odds and to fill her life with an important purpose.

Both Vinni's parents died of cancer shortly after she was married. Within five years her sister was diagnosed, as her mother had been, with breast cancer. Then, just three short years after her sister's diagnosis, Vinni, too, learned that she had metastatic breast cancer. She could have given up, resigned to the fact that, like her parents, this was a war she wasn't going to win. But not Vinni.

A self-described fighter, Vinni said she had three wonderful reasons to fight: her husband, Michael, and her two young sons, Christopher and Nicholas, who needed her. Determined to conquer the cancer, she endured several surgeries, including a bilateral mastectomy, and six difficult months of chemotherapy. Months of counseling, support groups, a change in diet and exercise, and the love of her family all worked together to get her through what she calls the most grueling period of her life.

"One night I kissed my children and put them to bed looking like the mother they knew. The next morning they woke up and I had no hair," she recalls. The effects of chemotherapy had begun. Fatigue, weight gain and loss, nausea, vomiting, pain, and susceptibility to illness slowed her physically, but mentally she never lost sight of her goal to get well.

In the early stages of her treatment, she devoted a great deal of her strength to trying to make herself look as best as possible. "Some days I'd see my reflection in the mirror and wonder who it was. I had always been healthy looking—now I was bald, bloated, and pale. I remember thinking I didn't want to scare my children—but they were so loving that every one of their responses just made me feel better."

She found wigs, learned to tie scarves in creative ways to hide her baldness, and used makeup to play up her beautiful eyes, despite the fact that her eyelashes and brows, too, had disappeared. "Makeup and hairpieces became very important to me. How I looked was about the only thing in my life that I had some control over—everything else was in the hands of the doctors. They told me what to do, how to think and eat. With my appearance I had a few choices. Knowing that got me through a terrible phase."

Today her cancer is in remission.

Convinced that a positive mind-set was key to her recovery, Vinni decided to concentrate on helping other cancer victims to feel encouraged. "I know that I felt best on the days when I was feeling feminine, pretty, and pampered—it helped me, that's all I can say."

With that in mind, Vinni founded her own company, "Beauté, Cancer and Having Style," a service devoted to providing cancer patients with a few hours of luxury and comfort, a form of care that is between medical therapy and family support. Facials, manicures, pedicures, and makeup lessons are all part of the service she provides. Best of all, she is able to answer questions and respond from her own experience to the personal feelings of women stricken with this frightening disease. "When you are ill, you are filled with fear and loneliness," she explains. "I want to help alleviate those emotional pains for other women.

"There was a time when I took all of life's wonders for granted, but not anymore," Vinni says now. "Someday when I die, I want God to look at me and say He was grateful He gave me a second chance."

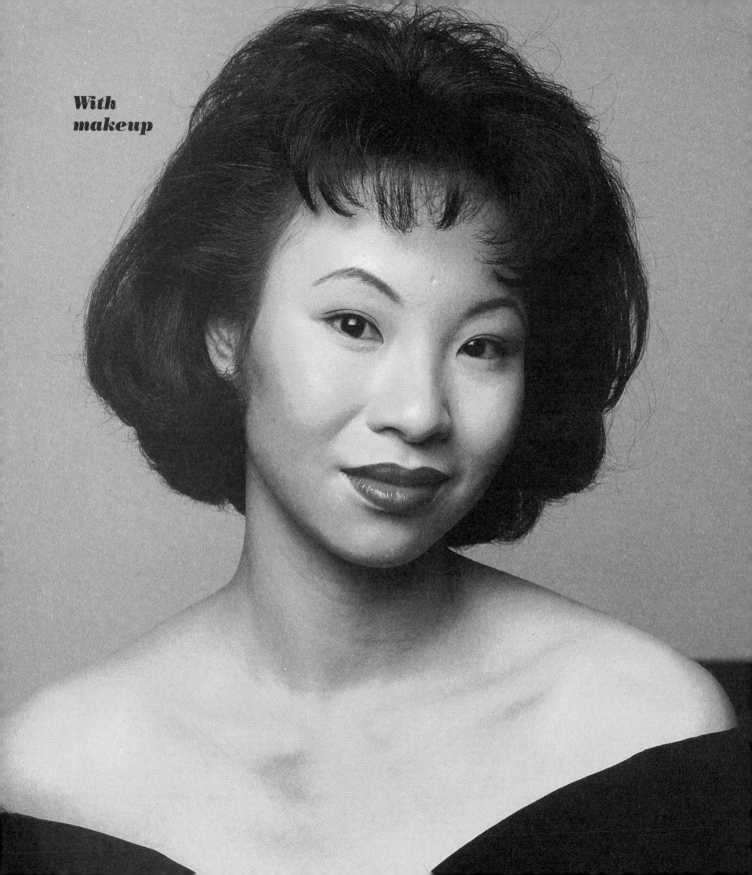

With
makeup

Wendy Fang Chen

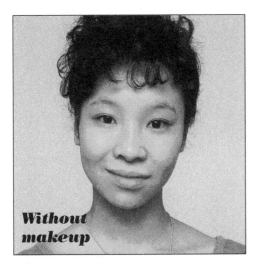

Without makeup

When Wendy Fang Chen was four and one-half years old her career as a pianist had begun. Her mother, who also had played the piano since childhood, recognized Wendy's natural musical talent. Nurturing her child's creative side, Mrs. Chen tutored the little girl at the piano. By the time Wendy turned seven, she was accepted into the precollege division of the Juilliard School, and by eight she was already composing. At eleven she had been on television, lauded in newspapers, and performed at Carnegie Recital Hall. There was no arguing that this gifted young artist deserved the label child prodigy.

As a teenager she maintained a full schedule of regular school, where she was an honor student, in addition to her specialized studies at Juilliard. Her life was filled with more concerts, publicity, radio and television interviews, and honors. Her music echoed through Lincoln Center in New York, the Kennedy Center in Washington, D.C., and various concert halls in Japan and Taiwan. She also conducted and organized the precollege composers chorus at Juilliard. It would have been quite a full life for any adult, yet she was still in high school.

"I matured fast because I dealt with a lot of older people—I was friends with teachers at school because I had known most of them for many years. My classmates and teachers respected me in a way that isn't usually bestowed on a child," Wendy recalls.

But as Wendy began to mature, being the "child" star brought some baggage with it. "In terms of my music, I was treated like an adult because I played like one. But, personally, even when I was a teenager, I still felt like a kid in many ways. Many people still regarded me as a 'child star' in the classical music world." She remembers asserting her young adulthood for the first time at sixteen. She appeared on stage in her first sophisticated dress: a strapless red gown that she had chosen all by herself. Teachers in her audience gasped.

"They were whispering that I wasn't a little girl anymore. I already knew that I was growing up, but people around me had to start rethinking their image of me. People didn't want to let go of the thought of me as a child, because in some ways it was more impressive that such a young person could play so well. But I was definitely growing up; my body and mind were changing."

When she entered the world-renowned Juilliard music school as a full-time college student, Wendy's life changed dramatically. She recognized that this was a turning point in her personal and professional life. Despite the fact that she had been named to the prestigious group of this country's presidential scholars and had been interviewed on national television programs as one of the most academically and artistically talented high school graduates in the United States, she had trepidations about college.

"I had always been at the top, the best at what I did. Now I was surrounded by the best of the best from all over the world—from Russia, Japan, and Korea. I was starting college and had to prove myself all over again," she recalls.

During those college years Wendy decided it was time to take charge of her own life. "I don't know if it was a conscious decision to 'become an adult'—when do you become an adult?—but I did start taking responsibility for myself. I moved out of my parents' home, started paying my own bills, and made my own decisions—that was something I never had really done before."

With her increasing confidence, she chose to leave behind the image of prodigy. The child-star presence that she had always assumed on stage changed. Though she maintained the natural look that she preferred, she experimented with more intense makeup colors, sophisticated hairstyles, and high-style gowns. The ingenue who appeared in one concert in February of 1991 emerged as a confident, gifted woman at her Carnegie Hall debut in May of that same year. "I still remember how big the [Carnegie] recital hall seemed to me when I was eleven—being in the main concert hall at Carnegie Hall as an adult caused the same thrill."

Today, at twenty-three, Wendy does her own hair and makeup before every performance. "I feel more comfortable when I look like myself, rather than someone else's idea of what I should look like," she explains. During the rigorous practice schedules that precede each concert, she maintains her privacy and takes long, relaxing baths to de-stress her body and her mind. "Now that I'm the one taking care of my life and my career, I'm much more aware and responsible. Now I know if I don't do well, everyone is going to witness it. As a child I was never aware of the consequences. I'm very serious about my work."

But at the same time, Wendy is determined to "have a life—a lot of former child prodigies don't have a personal life." She makes an effort to develop her whole self, not just the career side. "Instead of constant practice, I do things that make me a well-rounded person and enhance my playing. I have a boyfriend, I go to movies and comedy clubs, I work on my computer as a hobby, and I write."

Wendy took the initiative to add the balance she thought was missing. She began traveling around the world for her concerts on her own ("My mother had always accompanied me before"), encountering all the problems that child stars are often shielded from. And finding her own ways of handling them.

In facing adulthood, she seems to have developed some important perspective as well:

"I'm twenty-three and I'm doing the same job I've done since I was seven. Now I know that if I didn't love it, I wouldn't do it. The thrill of performing on stage is still there for me. It's so wonderful. My great joy now comes from filling my life with music. I won't be disappointed if I'm not the primo star in the world—I just want to keep performing. And of course I want to be happy. That's what's most important to me."

In my book, that makes her a primo star already. By the way, she already has recorded her first CD with the London Philharmonic Orchestra, on which she plays a piano concerto that she composed. We'll be hearing lots more from Wendy as her career continues to soar.

Be Your Own Role Model

16

66**Women who live for the next miracle cream do not realize that beauty comes from a secret happiness and equilibrium within themselves.**99

—Sophia Loren

Other people's achievements can be an inspiration—that's why role models are so important. But the key to increasing our self-esteem is our own positive action. When we *do* things that we're proud of, no matter how big or small, we feel better about ourselves.

Throughout this book I've offered my ideas about how using makeup can start a positive chain reaction. But remember: it all hinges on you. What you do every day can improve your life. In these last few pages, I want to share some of the ways I've learned to make positive things happen in my life. They have very little to do with lip-

153

> **"Where is the love, beauty and truth we seek/But in our mind?"**
>
> —Percy Bysshe Shelley

> **"It's a good thing that beauty is only skin deep, or I'd be rotten to the core."**
>
> —Phyllis Diller

stick and eyeshadow, yet they have everything to do with looking in the mirror and liking what I see.

These days I try to be my own role model. I make a concerted effort to be the best that I can be, whatever I'm doing. I am honest with myself. I challenge myself. I compete with myself and no one else. Above all, I accept myself. That's not to say that I don't try to change and try to improve. But I've learned that I cannot change what I have not yet accepted. Unless I am absolutely objective about myself and ready to acknowledge that "this is who I am and this is how I am behaving right now," I can't make positive changes. That goes for very simple things like trying out a new hairdo or style of makeup, or much more complex matters such as venturing into a business deal, or, as I did very recently, committing my life to a new person, getting married, and expanding our family.

One of the questions I ask myself often is "What is best for me?" For many years I couldn't ask that question—it felt too selfish. After all, I would tell myself, I have the needs of many other people in my life to think about. I finally realized, however, that when I carefully thought about that important question—What's best for me?—the answer often turned out to be the best for those around me as well as for myself. Now I have enough self-esteem to believe that when I'm happy about my life, it makes my family's and friends' lives happier, too. Conversely, when each person in my family is content, I feel content. Being happy and doing what is best for ourselves isn't a selfish pursuit, but a gift we share.

When I decide to take actions to improve my situation, I accept the responsibility for my actions. That way, I know that I have made a difference in my own life. Instead of returning to my old passive ways, I find being an active participant in my own future makes me feel powerful. It makes me trust myself. And, most important, it makes me like myself better.

To achieve those things that I determine are best for me, I set goals. Some are lofty (I remember when starting a cosmetics company seemed like an almost impossible goal), some are tiny (the car needs to be washed every week—I feel better when my car is clean). Some are very long

> **"Beauty is a pledge of the possible conformity between the soul and nature, and consequently a ground of faith in the supremacy of the good."**
>
> —George Santayana

> **"Beauty as we feel it is something indescribable: what it is or what it means can never be said."**
>
> —George Santayana

range (yes, I've already started saving for my four-month-old daughter's college education—I don't want the pressure later on), some very short term (I've got to call today to make an appointment for my next haircut—I hate waking up to a bad-hair day). They're all important to some aspect of my life.

When a goal is a decided challenge, I use visualization as a tool to achieve it. I cultivate an image in my mind and keep focusing on that abstraction until it becomes a reality. Visualization has been an important part of my process of becoming who I am, especially at times when a particular change isn't inherently natural. I visualize the change and amplify the idea in my mind before I own it completely. For instance, when I first started trying to build my business, my self-esteem was pretty low, I was nervous and sometimes wondered if I could achieve what I had set out to do.

I understood that I needed to feel more positive, but developing my own self-confidence was still very much a work in progress. So I began visualizing what a woman with very high self-esteem would think like, sound like, dress like, and act like. Whenever I could I would focus on a female image that was analytical, powerful, quick on her feet, sophicated, direct. Inside I still felt shy and quiet. But I persevered with the visualization, planting the image of that successful woman in my brain. Within a relatively short time I realized I was living that image. Today I am—generally—a confident businesswoman. And when those feelings falter—and yes, my level of self-esteem goes up and down—I visualize the image I want and quickly regain my composure.

Maybe understanding visualization explains why makeup helps us feel better about ourselves. There's a parallel between visualization and wearing cosmetics. In both we envision how great we can be. And with both self-help methods, the end result is that we improve our image. A new, enhanced look comes from the makeup. And a new, enhanced self-image comes along with the visualization. Ultimately we've created them ourselves. And with each new day we become more comfortable with both.

You'll notice that as your self-esteem increases,

66The saying that beauty is but skin deep is a skin-deep saying.99

—Herbert Spencer

66We are born with one face, but, laughing or crying, wisely or unwisely, eventually we form our own.99

—Coco Chanel

157

your positive feelings about the image you see in the mirror will increase in geometric proportions. You're probably not going to look dramatically different. No, the big change is going to be how you see yourself. You'll see your personal best—your true, true beauty. And I know you'll like what you see.

I know you're on the road to personal success. I'd love to hear about the route you take and the changes you make. Write and let me know how it goes. Best of luck!

Love,

Victoria

P.S. You can write to me at 8205 Santa Monica Blvd., #1-210, Los Angeles, CA 90046.

P.P.S. For more information about my products you can call toll-free 800-V-MAKEUP. I'd love for you to try them. But remember, you can follow the steps in this book using any brand of makeup.

66*Once upon a time, I was beautiful. My hair was thick and dark and glossy. My skin was smooth and soft as a ripe peach...my mouth was dark pink...my eyes were large and clear... Unfortunately, I was four years old at the time. It's been downhill ever since.*99

—Geneen Roth

A Special Thank You

On the next two pages are the 22 exceptional women who helped me redefine beauty in the pages of this book. Working with them was an extraordinary honor for me, as I discovered their inner beauty and personal accomplishments as well as their good looks. As you can see, each is uniquely attractive with makeup AND without. No picture has been retouched, so you can see the women exactly as they are: truly beautiful. I salute these remarkable models for appreciating and enhancing their individual beauty, and for confidently allowing me to use their faces for the natural-look makeup demonstrations in these pages. Each one of them, like you, is very special to me.

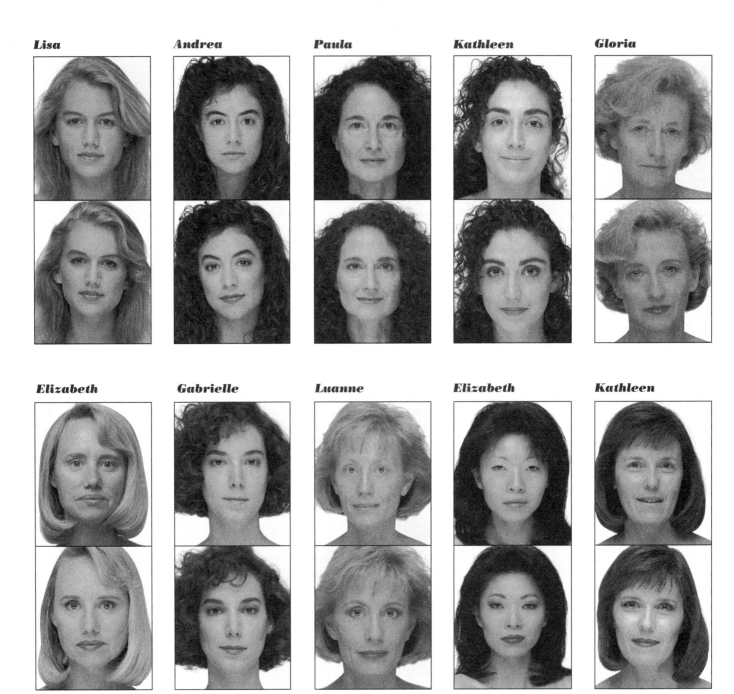

Lisa

Andrea

Paula

Kathleen

Gloria

Elizabeth

Gabrielle

Luanne

Elizabeth

Kathleen

Camey

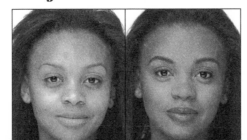

Sydney

Jaclyn

Wendy

Sibel

Kaoru

Carol

Trish

Kristen

Lisa

Laura

Roberta

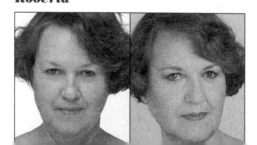

161